Viktor E. Frankl Goes to Community College

Health Communication

Gary L. Kreps, Series Editor

Vol. 18

The Health Communication series is part of
the Peter Lang Media and Communication list.
Every volume is peer reviewed and meets
the highest quality standards for content and production.

PETER LANG
New York • Bern • Berlin
Brussels • Vienna • Oxford • Warsaw

Janet Farrell Leontiou

Viktor E. Frankl Goes to Community College

How Creating Meaning May Save Your Life

PETER LANG
New York • Bern • Berlin
Brussels • Vienna • Oxford • Warsaw

Library of Congress Cataloging-in-Publication Control Number: 2021053846

Bibliographic information published by **Die Deutsche Nationalbibliothek**.
Die Deutsche Nationalbibliothek lists this publication in the "Deutsche Nationalbibliografie"; detailed bibliographic data are available on the Internet at http://dnb.d-nb.de/.

ISSN 2153-1277
ISBN 978-1-4331-8625-7 (hardcover)
ISBN 978-1-4331-8633-2 (paperback)
ISBN 978-1-4331-8626-4 (ebook pdf)
ISBN 978-1-4331-8627-1 (epub)
DOI 10.3726/b19263

80 Broad Street, 5th floor, New York, NY 10004
www.peterlang.com

For my boys, Zach and Andreas.
And…in loving memory of James Farrell.

Contents

Acknowledgments

A student once asked: "When did you begin teaching the course through the lens of logostherapy?" It was so long ago that I do not recall a time when I was not teaching logostherapy. I do know that I constructed the theory with the intention of giving something to my students that was meaningful for them. I never imagined that I would end up teaching at a community college. Looking back, I now see that I was exactly where I was supposed to be.

I am grateful that I was able to do my work over a span of twenty-seven years and counting. None of it would have been possible without my students' magnificent receptivity. I have always understood that it was their choice to listen and to learn that made all things possible. I never took that for granted.

The classroom can be an organic, creative, and exciting place. I hope that I was able to capture some of that dynamism on these pages and the reader can imagine how these ancient ideas may be able to shift us to a new place.

Introduction

I have spent the last twenty-seven years teaching my adapted version of Frankl's logotherapy to community college students. Frankl's theory of logotherapy is a psychotherapy based on meaning. I chose, those many years ago, to develop the course because I agree with Frankl that a life without meaning is not sustainable. Frankl makes the point exceedingly clear that many mental health issues such as depression, aggression, addictions and some suicides can be linked back to the sufferer experiencing a lack of meaning.[1] In Frankl's words: "As to the causation of the feeling of meaninglessness, one may say, albeit in an oversimplifying vein, that people have enough to live by but nothing to live for; they have the means but no meaning."[2]

The topic of suicide was always at the forefront of Frankl's work. Before he was imprisoned by the Nazis, his psychiatric research focused on trying to understand the increase in suicides among students during report card distribution. We are told that he framed the

1 Viktor E. Frankl, *Man's Search for Meaning* (Boston: Beacon Press, 2006), 107.
2 Frankl, 140.

entire psychiatric encounter by asking the patient: "Why do you not commit suicide?"[3] He did this because he knew if could help patients identify their reason for living and to acknowledge what they are living for, they would be less likely to take their own lives. Frankl tells us: "A man who becomes conscious of the responsibility he bears toward a human being who affectionately waits for him, or an unfinished work, will never be able to throw his life away."[4] Here, Frankl is telling us that it is our love and work (two parts of the trilogy of logotherapy) are what gives our lives meaning. The work we need to do as human beings is to figure out how love and work fit within the context of our own lives. Frankl borrows some of his theoretical framework from the philosopher, Friedrich Nietzsche, who said: "He who has a *why* to live for can bear with any *how*."[5]

The Existentialists, and the Stoics who preceded them, understood that life does not come with a pre-established meaning and if our lives are meaningless, it is because we have not put the meaning into our lives. We are the ones who need to do the necessary work of constructing meaning. Sometimes people, especially young people, fall into despair and they choose to end their lives before they do the necessary work. If they could have endured the pain a bit longer, they may have been able to arrive at a new place of understanding. Frankl tells us that whenever he was confronted with a person who was prone to suicide, he reports what others have told him in the past.

> I explain to such a person that patients have repeatedly told me how happy they were that the suicide attempt had not been successful; weeks, months, years later, they told me, it turned out that there was a solution to their problem, an answer to their question, a meaning to their life.[6]

Frankl's entire thesis is based upon how a strong orientation toward constructing meaning within one's life plays an essential role in the prevention of suicide.

3 Gordon W. Allport's preface in Viktor E. Frankl's *Man's Search for Meaning* (New York: Simon & Schuster, 1959), 9.
4 Frankl, *Man's Search for Meaning* (Boston: Beacon Press, 2006), 80.
5 Frankl, *Man's Search for Meaning* (Boston: Beacon Press, 2006), 76.
6 Frankl, *Man's Search for Meaning* (Boston: Beacon Press, 2006), 142.

We are now living through a pandemic that has wreaked havoc with our lives. Frankl's words, as well as the Stoic philosophy that inspired them, have become especially poignant during these challenging times. A few of the Stoic themes that are especially useful right now are: what happens to us is outside of our realm of control, the only thing we can choose is our response, to live is to suffer, and our work is to discover the meaning in the suffering.

If we take Frankl at his word, we can discover that there is the potential to become better people for having suffered through a pandemic. Of course, no one chooses to suffer and if given the choice, we would choose to forego this experience but we are not given the choice. It is all outside the realm of our control. The only choice we have is how we choose to see our experience. The only sensible choice toward reality is to accept it since things will not change simply because we wish it to change. We are the ones who need to change, and herein lies our power.

Frankl made it out of the camp alive. He was not killed by the Nazis, and he did not "run into the wire" or kill himself. In his book he left us a guide in the form of a love letter outlining precisely how we too cannot only survive this life but create a meaningful life and use our suffering to take us to an even better place in our lives. Now, during the pandemic, we are poised at a moment in time to create meaning. Frankl tells us: "Man is capable of changing the world for the better if possible, and of changing himself for the better if necessary."[7]

The chapters are broken down into understanding how Frankl is instructing us in becoming agents of change within our own lives. As you read the chapters, I invite you to see how Frankl's life was informed by the ideas I have highlighted here and to imagine how the ideas may come to change and shape how you see your own life.

I begin with the Stoics because Frankl's book could not have been written without his knowledge of this ancient wisdom. In my teaching, I stress that ideas and words are handed down to us. Etymologically, the word *tradition* means to hand down. These words, however, are not dead but require that we infuse them with new life. This is what Frankl did by creating logotherapy from Stoicism. This is what I did by

7 Frankl, *Man's Search for Meaning* (Boston: Beacon Press, 2006), 131.

creating logostherapy from logotherapy. This is what I encourage my students to do.

Many of the ideas presented in *Man's Search for Meaning,* at first seem counter- cultural and may even sound counter-intuitive. For instance, he tells us to develop an attitude of being outwardly focused on the world and on others. He is telling us that the best way to develop as human beings is not to focus on the self but instead to reach out and help others to develop within their own lives. I realize that if you are depressed and lack enthusiasm for your own life, this request may sound impossible, but it need not be a grand gesture. A small gesture such as checking- in on a friend may become the start of a shift.

What Frankl is asking for (although he never uses the word) is what the Greeks would call a metanoia or a complete change of mind. This change of mind holds that retreating into oneself is ultimately not in one's own best interest. I think that it cannot be overstated that this outward focus is a central theme within Frankl's book. The places within the book when Frankl speaks of a change in attitude, he is specifically speaking about a shift from inward focus to outward focus.

When we engage in this metanoia, it changes how we see all the aspects of our lives—our mental health, our speech, our suffering, our love, and our work. If I read Frankl correctly, the reason why we often are so unsuccessful in these domains within our lives is because of our approach. In many ways, the way in which we have constructed our lives directly pushes against that which Frankl has outlined. Therefore, I see his claims as radical.

His radicalness, however, is not in forging a new path but instead he is putting us back on an old path from which we strayed. One of the old paths is the religious concept that it is better to give than receive. The understanding contained within the ancient wisdom is that the only way we receive anything within our lives is when we give expecting nothing in return. This perspective is consistent with the advice sometimes offered to those feeling down. Step out and start small but see what you may be able to offer another. The giving is not so that you will see that there are others who suffer more greatly than you. I have always disliked that line of thought for several reasons. One, as Frankl states within the book, everyone's suffering is legitimate for its own sake and comparison/contrast has nothing to do with suffering because suffering cannot be quantified or measured.[8] Two, I strongly dislike using another's misfortune to evoke gratitude for one's own life. That seems to me to be selfishly using another person's circumstances of life for one's own personal gain. For example, I have a child who uses a wheelchair and I do not want him to be used to make other children feel grateful that they have legs (and arms) that work. Instead, I would rather see kindness expressed to him simply because one can and expecting nothing in return. It is only then that we will see that we will receive in ways we hardly imagine. Once our expectations enter the picture, it clouds the intention and thwarts the potential to receive.

Let's, for a moment, bring this idea of expectation back to how we expect our lives to unfold. It is not the unfolding of our lives that is the problem but instead the problem comes from the inability to let go of the notion that our lives will unfold according to our expectations. I immediately recognize the arrogance of that stance. Frankl asks that we not only recognize the arrogance but also understand that suffering, while not what we expect nor want, may just be what we most need.

Frankl's book was written about his time spent within several Nazi German concentration camps. These are the lessons he brought back to us from lived experience. His book is not written to document the atrocities the Germans committed against the Jews. There are other books to serve that function for documenting historical records. Frankl's book, instead, asks us to reflect upon how we are choosing to live our own lives by showing us how he chose to reflect upon his own. He came by this insight the hard way—from circumstances outside his realm of control. He came upon this insight when his life was stripped bare of all that made it recognizable. What I think he was left with was the essential truth and it is that truth he is offering us.

This little book of mine is meant to serve as a companion piece to Frankl's. What I offer is twenty-seven years of experience bringing these teachings to community college students. Over the years, I have had a front seat in observing students engage with the metanoia that not only resulted in them changing their minds but also changing their lives.

8 Frankl, *Man's Search for Meaning* (Boston: Beacon Press, 2006), 44.

Just as Frankl had an intention concerning what kind of book he wished to write, I also have my own agenda in writing this book. This book does not aim to provide historical nor psychological context. Those areas are not my expertise. I am also not very interested to rehash how scholars have received Frankl's theories. What does interest me, and where I hope that I have something useful to say, is sharing with you the context I have created for this book for my students. The context consists of both the roots and wings of Frankl's theory. In other words, I choose to stress the roots of Stoicism within logotherapy in addition to the wings of my theory of logostherapy.

My work, at its essence, is about words—specifically, it is recovering the power of the spoken word. Frankl has created a theory of logotherapy—of creating a meaningful life. The task of creating a meaningful life cannot, in my opinion, be accomplished until we begin to see words differently than we see them currently. On the list of what we have forgotten, the power of words tops the list. Logostherapy, when broken down into its Greek origins, means attending to the word.

We seem to subscribe to the myth that words are insignificant things. We have many maxims within the culture that reinforce the inadequacy of words. I have always thought that putting down words is not good for us. I have learned, from teaching my students, to see words differently is the catalyst to seeing the entire world differently. We hear people occasionally attempt to redeem words by saying "words matter." After reading this book, my wish is that the reader not only understands that words absolutely matter but also understands how they matter and why they matter.

The word *myth* comes from the Greek mythos—meaning a telling. Myth, contrary to popular belief, is not something false but instead a myth is what we recreate through our words—it is what we say. It could be true, or it could be false. Take, for instance, the myth of the self-made man. This myth is, I think, always false because no one can make it without the help of others. Frankl was able to make it out alive because he knew the teachings from the Stoics and he experienced love from his wife, family, and fellow prisoners. Sometimes, my students think that what they have accomplished, they accomplished on their own. Part of my work is to have them see that is usually never true. For instance,

I remember a conversation with a student who had graduated from a severely under-performing high school that has a 50% graduation rate. I asked her how it was that she made it out, was able to graduate, and was able to attend college? Was there someone within the high school that helped her? She then told me that there was one guidance counselor who checked up on a group of students. He was the one who made sure that the students did their work and attended class. I think that it is possible for the student to overlook the importance of this counselor within her life, and I think that if the student believes that she did it on her own, she will be less likely to reach out a hand to others. The truth is rarely does anyone make it on his or her own but instead the person needs to be invited to start to see all the ways that he or she has been helped by others. On the flip side of deconstructing this myth is the awareness that if you are struggling within your life right now, you need not go it alone.

References

Note: The edition of Frankl's book that is used here, unless otherwise noted, is: Viktor E. Frankl, *Man's Search for Meaning*. Boston: Beacon Press, 2006.

Allport, Gordon W. Preface. Viktor E. Frankl's *Man's Search for Meaning*. New York: Simon & Schuster, 1959.

Frankl, Viktor E. *Man's Search for Meaning*. Boston: Beacon Press, 2006.

Chapter One

The Stoics

All the overt references to Stoic philosophy have been scrubbed from Frankl's book. While I understand the editorial choice, I do not agree. I was once advised to remove the theoretical framework from one of my books by the editor because the thought was that the theory would bog down the book and limit readership. When I read Frankl, I see the influence of the Stoics but my students do not. I think that the choice to edit out the connection to Stoicism makes it seem like the book merely sprung from Frankl's head.

I tell my students that the book sprang from the fact that Frankl had already received an education upon entering the camps. More importantly, the education that Frankl had received in philosophy, more so than in psychology, was that which saved his life. This is an important point to make when we live in a time where job skills are emphasized within school and the liberal arts are under constant attack. I stress that a liberal arts education may provide you with that which is necessary to build a life. My students, I think, need to hear this message and it is one I have been delivering for the last twenty-seven years although the message is rarely supported by influences outside the classroom.

The foundation for Stoicism came from Zeno, born 490 B.C. Zeno found himself shipwrecked and without resources. He had lost everything and through that loss, built an entire system of philosophy that still resonates today. We can immediately begin to see the points of intersection between Zeno and Frankl. Zeno began to teach his theory from a porch-like structure (the word Stoic comes from the portico where school was taught) and he began to acquire followers. Once we understand the anchoring of this philosophy, we see that Frankl adopted every single one of them and breathed into them new life.

Stoicism taught Frankl that while we cannot choose what happens to us, we can choose how it is that we respond to what happens to us. This deceptively simple sounding statement is probably the most difficult to master. The Stoics talked about developing the discernment to learn the difference between what is within our control and what is not. The Stoics, then, provide us with a guide to avoid driving ourselves insane by resisting and/or trying to change that which is not in our power to change. This response really sums up Frankl's situation within the camp. He was a prisoner within the concentration camp and no amount of wishful thinking will change that fact. Here is what I have come to understand as the life-long undertaking of the process of acceptance. Everyone has circumstances within his or her life that just are. My circumstance is that I have a child with disability. This is just a factual reality of my life. Anything other than acceptance does not produce positive outcomes for him or for me. I have come to learn that acceptance is anything but one and done. Acceptance is a life-long process that needs to be revisited time and time again. This is especially clear for me as my son has a typically developing twin brother and as milestones are reached, acceptance needs to constantly be revisited. Also, the type of acceptance I am talking about is not complacent but instead a very engaged, active process.

The next hurdle to take on is the choice to not only accept but to see that all we have been given is a gift. This is not the gift we were expecting to receive but a gift, nonetheless. I think this inherent optimism within the Stoic philosophy may influence the denotation of the word stoic to describe someone who has equanimity—not deflated by the lows and not elated by the highs. The ancient Stoic saw everything we have been given as a gift from the gods and developed the discipline to receive all with a welcoming and trusting heart.

The Stoic philosophy is inherently practical since it teaches that since we cannot change reality, why not adapt to reality and use it as an opportunity to grow? Frankl came into the camps working on a book about suicide and found himself in a situation to fully understand why people choose to take their own lives. Life, sometimes, when looked at through this lens of Stoicism gives us exactly what we most need but what we would never choose. As we will come to see, Frankl made the internal decision to continue his work within the camps and that internal choice had a major impact upon his survival.

Upon entering the concentration camp, Frankl lost his freedom and his life as he knew it. There was nothing he could do about changing this truth. In addition to this major loss upon entering the camp, he also lost his manuscript (his mental child) and there was nothing he could do except accept that fact as well. Like the Stoic he was, he understood what was within his realm of control and what was not. Also, he looked to see the opportunities present in what he was given—as incredibly difficult as that must have been.

Although nothing like Frankl's circumstances, I have attempted to emulate both him and the Stoics who informed him. Last year, while in a pandemic lock-down, the opportunity presented itself to create a podcast on Frankl with a woman who lived in Brazil. A third party introduced us, and this third party was to be the executive producer of the podcast. My co-host and I worked extremely hard to create the content for this podcast and had created all that was required in bringing the podcast to market. I wrote the scripts for both of us and my co-host handled the technical aspects of the podcast. We recorded and edited the shows, created the content, opened the social platforms, and created the website. The executive producer, around the time of our official launch, disappeared. I wanted to move on without him but because he was the financial backer of the project, my co-host decided to back away. She refused to talk to me, and she began to take down all that we had publicly posted. There was nothing I could do about the decisions made by either the producer or the co-host. Both were outside of the realm of my control. The idea for the writing of this book was born within the context of the destruction of the podcast. Adopting a Stoic mindset, which is extremely optimistic and hopeful, is to see that all the work I put into that podcast as the preparation necessary to write this book. Adopting a Stoic mentality is choosing to trust that all is for the good and all unfolds as it is supposed to unfold.

In addition to acceptance, Frankl developed his framework from the Stoic idea of radical freedom and radical responsibility. I tell my students that I can open the book at random and the passage will be about choice because the entire book is about choice. I am free to make any choice I wish and everything I do or say is my choice. However, for every choice, I am accountable. Frankl instructs us that the terms of liberty and responsibility are correlative terms. There is no such thing as freedom without responsibility. I think that we need to hear this message since sometimes we wish to have the freedoms but not the responsibilities that go along with the liberties. Frankl states that in the US, we should have a statue of responsibility on the West Coast to balance the statue of liberty on the East Coast:

"In fact, freedom is in danger of degenerating into mere arbitrariness unless it is lived in terms of responsibleness."[1]

Another essential idea that Frankl takes from the Stoics is that to live is to suffer. Suffering is part of the human condition. People sometimes feel that they are all alone in their suffering and this is both true and not true. People's suffering is within the context of their own lives and no two people suffer in the same way. The way in which I suffer is particular to me but I may be able to gain comfort from knowing that indeed everyone does suffer. Sometimes people ask: "why me?" but within the Stoic framework, the question becomes: "Why not me?" Suffering is what we humans share and knowing that is comforting. As you will come to read in the following pages, I believe in the generative power of words and that speaking creates community. Once I start to speak about my experience, usually others start to speak of their experience and then I may be able to experience community instead of isolation.

1 Frankl, 132.

All these ideas, borrowed from Stoicism, were that which Frankl used to develop his theory of logotherapy. Gordon Allport did refer to Frankl's theory as a philosophy and not as a psychology.[2] Allport is the only one who mentions, within his preface to Frankl's book, Frankl's Stoic/existential roots.[3] Maybe the greatest connection between Frankl and Zeno is the reference to the logos. Frankl called his theory logotherapy from the Greek word the logos, which Frankl states denotes meaning. This comment is somewhat misleading in Frankl. The word *logos* in Greek does not have a one-word English translation. Zeno, in creating his philosophy, also begins with the logos and Frankl follows him. The way in which Zeno used it implied the divine reason implicit in the cosmos, ordering it and giving it form as well as meaning. The way in which I understand logos is that it is both found in the world and within us. One thing is clear: logos is much bigger than human reason. Frankl constantly circles back to this way of looking at meaning as much bigger than our own small realm of reference within our own lives. Therefore the concept of the logos is tricky. The logos is our personal meaning within a context that is bigger than us.

I will return to the concept of the logos within the next chapter because I have created my own theory of logostherapy as inspired by Frankl's theory of logotherapy. I think that once we understand that logotherapy is Stoicism but is just called something different, we begin to see that ideas do not grow within a vacuum but instead ideas morph and take on other forms. This is my argument against editing out the explicit references to Stoicism within the book. Instead, I teach my students that ideas (and words, also, as the next chapter will demonstrate), have an ancestry and a legacy. All ideas come from somewhere and they go somewhere. The philosophy of Stoicism later informed the philosophy of existentialism and within Frankl's hands, informed logotherapy. Ideas have both roots and wings. I teach my students about the Stoic and existential roots of logotherapy. I also demonstrate how Frankl provided me with my own wings to create my own theory of

2 Gordon Allport preface in Viktor E. Frankl, *Man's Search for Meaning* (New York: Simon & Schuster, Inc., 1959), 11.

3 Allport, 12.

logostherapy. My students take these lessons to heart. One student gave a talk about how she never understood that she was, indeed, a Stoic in temperament. She now has a word to connect her experience to that which is so much larger than her. Other students developed their own theory of listening by giving them permission to create and through offering theory generation as an option in class. All thinkers begin with previous accomplishment of thought and when I have pointed this out to students, it gives them permission to think.

The name Zeno is never mentioned within the book, but the name Nietzsche is mentioned and even when Nietzsche's name is not present, his ideas are central to the book. The references to Nietzsche and the use of the word "existential" throughout the book point to the presence of existential philosophy. Existentialism, however, is new wine in an old bottle. An existential philosopher like Nietzsche took the teachings of the ancient Stoics[4] and breathed into them new life in much the same way as Frankl did. When I teach students philosophy and the history of ideas, these teachings offer worthwhile content as to how to live their lives and models for them that sometimes "new" ways of seeing are, in fact, quite old. I remember learning, when I was a student, of the importance of wondering about origins. I remember learning that for the ancients, wondering about origins was the beginning of thought. Here I am talking about philosophical traditions but wondering about origins may pertain to anything: a word, our names, an expression, a thought, a theory, etc. Insight may come from following the path backwards to see how something came to be.

It is my wish that as you read this section on Stoicism, you come to understand that all the philosophers who labeled themselves Stoics and/or existentialists experienced tremendous pain within their personal lives. All of them created important, beautiful work from personal tragedy and brokenness. This is not to romanticize the image of the suffering artist but instead to emphasize the truth of what Nietzsche claimed (who was no foreigner to pain and suffering) that the most

4 For sure, there are differences between stoicism and existentialism. Some of Nietzsche's writings were critical of the Stoics but here, I am stressing the commonalities instead of the differences. Highlighting the points of intersection verses differences, like everything else, is the result of a choice.

glorious of human achievement is created from great suffering.[5] No one chooses to suffer and that is why Frankl carefully writes about "unavoidable" suffering. If you can avoid suffering, avoid it. There is no heroism or glory in becoming a masochist. But … if you cannot avoid it, work with it so that it may transform from something not chosen into a gift. Frankl tells us that through creating meaning from suffering, the suffering ceases to be suffering. In other words, he holds out the extraordinary possibility that everything may be for the good. This idea is found within the usual way that we use the word stoic to mean someone who does not show his or her feelings. The reason why the ancient Stoics did not become elated by the highs of life or deflated by the lows is because they chose to see that everything was a gift from the gods, and they strove toward creating the equanimity to receive all with gratitude.

Frankl is in good company with those thinkers who were inspired by the school of thought founded by Zeno. Men like Epictetus, Marcus Aurelius, and Seneca took up the baton passed down to them by Zeno. The one thing that all these men had in common is that they suffered greatly within their own personal lives. Zeno found himself shipwrecked, Epictetus was born a slave, Marcus Aurelius reigned over Rome during the time of a plague, and Seneca was exiled. It may be useful to take a closer look at the ideological commonplaces as well. A person who calls himself a Stoic possesses this set of qualities: has an accepting mindset toward reality, sees oneself as responsible, and acknowledges that one is free. Let's take another look at each of these three features to see how these ideas are connected to communication.

Accepting Reality

The great wisdom that the Stoics left us with is to develop the capacity to discern what is within our control and what is not. They understood that much of our misery comes from trying to control that which is not under our control. According to Epictetus, "The chief task in life

5 For an induction, see Leslie Paul Thiele, *Friedrich Nietzsche and the Politics of the Soul: A study of Heroic Individualism* (Princeton: Princeton University Press, 1990).

is simply this: to identify and separate matters so that I can say clearly to myself which are externals not under control, and which have to do with the choices I actually control."[6] This is the thought that inspired Frankl to formulate that it is our response to the situation that is the only thing within our realm of control and the only thing we can change is ourselves. According to one of Frankl's well-known statements: "When we are no longer able to change a situation—just think of an incurable disease such as inoperable cancer—we are challenged to change ourselves."[7]

To further clarify the Stoic understanding of acceptance, there is some nuance here. The Stoics are speaking about acceptance as a very active process and not a passive resignation. I can best explain by example. I have twin boys—one with disability and one typically developing. For each milestone my typical son reaches, I need to actively accept that his brother is in a very different place. They are now nineteen years old, and it has been like this for all their lives and will remain so for the rest of my life.

If there is one word that we use that represents the antithesis of an acceptance mindset, it is the word "should." Calling attention to how frequently we speak of a situation as it should be rather than how it is will reveal how much we are accepting (or not accepting) that which is out of our control. The word "should" implies that reality needs to conform to my expectations instead of my conforming to life. Within a Stoic framework, the only time "should" applies is when I choose to become what I know I should become. According to Marcus Aurelius: "Waste no more time arguing what a good man **should** be. Be one."[8] Frankl puts these words into practice when he speaks of the manuscript he lost upon entering the camps.

He needed to surrender his clothes and upon surrendering his coat, he surrendered the manuscript hidden within his coat. He was given a coat that most probably once belonged to another prisoner who had already been killed. He reflects on the experience like this:

6 Epictetus, *The Discourses as reported by Arrian, the Manual, and Fragments.* William Abbot, trans. (Charleston, SC: Nabu Press, 2018), 2.5.4–5.

7 Frankl, 112.

8 Marcus Aurelius *Meditations* (West Sussex, UK: John Wiley & Sons Ltd, 2020).

> Instead of the many pages of my manuscript, I found in a pocket of the newly acquired coat one single page torn out of a Hebrew prayer book, containing the most important Jewish prayer, *Shema Yisrael*. How should I have interpreted such a "coincidence" other than as a challenge to *live* my thoughts instead of merely putting them on paper?[9]

Within this quote, contains the element of responsibleness—another cornerstone of Stoicism and a cornerstone of Frankl's book. Listen for the echo of Epictetus within Frankl's point of view:

> Forces beyond your control can take everything you possess except one thing, your freedom to choose how you will respond to the situation. You cannot control what happens to you in your life, but you can always control what you will feel and do about what happens to you.[10]

I teach my students to discern the difference between responding and reacting. In responding, I imagine the options within my mind and choose the one that is most appropriate. Just because someone yells at me, does not mean that I need to yell back.

When I take that pause, I am remembering that I am free to choose another way. Responding is a result of thinking whereas reacting is usually kneejerk and the result of habit. If we are reacting, we are usually giving away our power and it is our reactions that mostly lead to feelings of regret. More damage is done, I think, from thoughtlessness than evil intentions. Most people do not wish to be hurtful, but their hurtfulness is the result of not thinking. When we respond, we become more response able (responsible).

I sometimes see those who attempt to make communication into a science and take a formulaic approach to communication. For instance, I have written two books about medical communication where I offer a critique of the approach to teaching doctors how to communicate by using a checklist and teaching communication as a skill.[11] Asking the

9 Frankl, 115.

10 This quote offered by Harold S. Kushner in Foreword to Viktor E. Frankl, *Man's Search for Meaning* (Boston: Beacon Press, 2006), X.

11 See Janet Farrell Leontiou, *The Doctor Still Knows Best: How Medical Culture is Still Marked by Paternalism* (New York: Peter Lang, 2020) and *What Do the Doctors Say?: How Doctors Create a World through Their Words* (Bloomington, IN: iUniverse, 2010).

patient or a family member a question because it is how one has been trained to talk is doomed to fail if the sincere intention is not present. This approach is the opposite of creating thoughtful communication. Communication cannot be turned into a formula because within every situation, all the variables change: who I become as the speaker, who my audience is, what is the message I wish to deliver as well as the context in which the communication occurs is constantly changing. Frankl reinforces this idea of the necessity of keeping in mind all the particularities of the situation: "No situation repeats itself and each situation calls for a different response."[12]

The final aspect of Stoicism that I wish to highlight is freedom. I have already written about Frankl's understanding that freedom and responsibility are correlative terms. One is meaningless without the other. There is a beautiful quote attributed to Frankl but as far I can tell, it may be more of Frankl's sentiment than his exact words: "Between stimulus and response there is a space. In our response lies our freedom and growth."[13] Freedom, then, is discovered in our capacity to pause; to stop and think how we wish to respond. Consider the habits of speech where we say that we are "forced" to do certain things, or we "have" to do certain things? This language imprisons us. In truth, we do not "have" to do anything and the only context in which the use of the word "force" is legitimate is within the context of violence. The other day, I was listening to a lawyer speak about violence as a communicative expression. Violence is not a communicative expression but instead is the decision to abandon communication. Violence is the choice to rob the other of their capacity to choose. Everything else is our choice.

The cornerstone of Zeno's philosophy of Stoicism is the logos. I think that Frankl was following Zeno in his choice to name his theory logotherapy. I do think that the Greek word *logos* is far more nuanced and complicated than Frankl lets on. One of the points I have attempted to make in the next chapter is how our words either free us or imprison us.

12 Frankl, 77.

13 I have been unable to locate this quote within Frankl although it is often attributed to him.

References

Allport, Gordon. Preface. Viktor E. Frankl, *Man's Search for Meaning.* New York: Simon & Schuster, 1959.

Aurelius, Marcus. *The Medications.* West Sussex, UK: John Wiley & Sons, 2020.

Epictetus. *The Discourses as reported by Arrian, the Manual and Fragments.* William Abbot, trans. Charleston, SC: Nabu Press, 2018.

Farrell Leontiou, Janet. *The Doctor Still Knows Best: How Medical Culture is Still Marked by Paternalism.* New York: Peter Lang, 2020.

———. *What Does the Doctor Say?: How Doctors Create a World through Their Words.* Indianapolis, IN: iUniverse, 2010.

Frankl, Viktor E. *Man's Search for Meaning.* Boston: Beacon Press, 2006.

Nietzsche, Friedrich. *Basic Writings of Nietzsche.* New York: Modern Library Classics, 2009.

Chapter Two

The Logos

I agree with Frankl that a meaningless life is not sustainable. The starting place for me is always how can we have meaning within our lives when we look upon words as meaningless? I think that over time, we have lost both the meaning of words and lost the understanding that words are powerful. I think that there has been a concerted effort to rob words of their meaning.

How did we arrive at this place of meaninglessness? I think that part of it goes back to the time when as a culture we transitioned from oral culture to written culture. It seems to me that prior to the invention of the written alphabet, people understood the power of the spoken word. Ancient peoples and oral cultures seemed to have understood the power of the spoken word. The ancients understood the power of the spoken word and anticipated the effects of the creation of the new technology, the written word, would have on us. Long before an understanding of neuroplasticity, Socrates warned us: "The alphabet will create forgetfulness in the learner's soul. They will trust the written characters and not remember themselves."[1]

Socrates understood that within an oral culture, each person was responsible for remembering and handing down the stories. Socrates was right that our memories have grown weaker over time, and we cannot imagine committing stories like *The Iliad* and *The Odyssey* to memory. Yet these stories existed as oral tales for generations before Homer wrote them down. In presenting the written alphabet as a technology, my students see the connection to their technologies and the impact their devices are having on them. There is no doubt that "We become what we behold. We shape our tools and then our tools shape us."[2]

I invite my students to think about their relationship with technology. Like everything else, the use of technology is both a benefit and a disadvantage. I have seen pedagogical discussions working from the general assumption that the more technology within the classroom, the better. The use of computers is more nuanced than that and nothing is a categorical good. My students are not readers of books. I describe them as being post-literate. They are not illiterate. They can read but it is just that they choose not to. When they do read, it is more often from a screen and not from the printed page of a book. Research tells us that the form does make a difference and that we tend to remember less when we read from a device.[3] The fact that my students read fewer books means that they have a different relationship with the written word. I recall that one student, for instance, pointed to a very straightforward passage in *Man's Search for Meaning* and commented: "He does not speak like we do." This passage contained no rhetorical flourishes nor any big words; I think that this comment is speaking to the

1 Plato, "Phaedrus," *Plato: Complete Works*, J.M.Cooper, ed. (Indianapolis IN: Hackett, 1997), 551–552.

2 This quote, often attributed to Marshall McLuhan, is from an article about McLuhan by Father John Culkin, "A Schoolman's Guide to Marshall McLuhan, *Saturday Review* (March 18, 1967), 70.

3 For some thoughts on the difference between reading from a screen versus reading from a page, see Ferris Jabr, "The Reading Brain in the Digital Age: The Science of Paper versus Screens," *Scientific American*, 11 April 2013. https://www.scientificamerican.com/article/reading-paper-science.

difference between written word and spoken word. The printed word is an unfamiliar technology for many of my students. It is for this reason that I teach a very close reading of the text.

I am now writing this book during a pandemic. Without the use of technology, we would be unable to hold class at all. I am very appreciative of the technology, and I think my students are as well. I am also raising a child who has disabilities. He is both non ambulatory and nonverbal. Without the technology, he cannot get around in the world nor communicate through words. He uses a wheelchair to get around and a communication eye gaze device to speak. Technology is a game changer for kids like mine.

My students end up loving Frankl's book; they get drawn into his story. I think that it is the story that hooks them. We are hardwired for story and narrative.[4] I teach every lesson using a story from my own personal life. I have found that students may forget explanations, but they will remember the story. The native American writer, Diane Glancy, states that "storying gives shape to meaning."[5] I love the grammatical shift she uses here to transform a noun into a verb. Speaking is not in opposition to action but is itself a form of action.

The expression "actions speak louder than words" creates a lot of damage and is but one of many expressions that downplay the power of spoken word. The old-fashioned maxim "sticks and stones may break my bones, but words will never hurt me" is untrue, not helpful, and may be producing the opposite of what we wish to create. The expression does not acknowledge the hurt and does not give the child strategies to act upon words that have hurt. Most importantly, the maxim gives tacit approval for children to do back to others what has been done to them. This is one way that we re-create the status quo and are complicit in the damage it creates.

4 See Lisa Cron, *Wired for Story: The Writer's Guide to Using Brain Science to Hook Readers from the Very First Sentence* (Berkeley, CA.: Ten Speed Press, 2012).

5 Diane Glancy, "Speaking The Corn into Being," in *The West Pole* (Minneapolis: University of Minnesota Press, 1997), 65–70. A version of this essay appeared in *The Utne Reader*, September 1, 1997, was where I first encountered it. I have been teaching this article for as long as I have been teaching. https://www.utne.com/mind-and-body/speaking-the-corn-into-being-cherokee-oral-tradition

The expression "those are nothing but words" sounds particularly nihilistic. I recall how a student spoke of a memory from school when a teacher used a bottle of Windex and cloth as a visual aid for the concept of ethnic cleansing. The student had the presence of mind to bring the issue to the principal only to be told that "those were just words." We also repeat the expression that "it is not what you say but how you say it" which is yet just another way to downplay words. Instead, it is both **what** you say and **how** you say it. Delivery cannot be separated from content.

I teach within the discipline of interpersonal communication and most textbooks within this discipline offer that meanings are not in words and words are arbitrary labels. I cannot think of anything more soul damaging than this way of thinking about words. Yet, it seems to be an accepted norm within the discipline. It was this understanding of language that is so very different from my own that motivated me to write my own textbook.[6] In my writing, etymology is at the forefront of my theory of communication.

Not knowing a word's etymology has resulted in words and meaning parting company. I think that once the teaching of Greek and Latin went out of fashion, so did etymology. If there is one thing that I teach that makes a difference within the student, it is learning a word's etymology. The etymology tells the story of the word and has a way to speak to us in a way that definition does not. The definition provides us with an abstract denotation, but it does not tell the story. As humans, we are inherently drawn to stories and the story stays with us. We remember stories. The difference between the etymology and denotation is the difference between story and explanation. The story invites us to discover the meaning for ourselves whereas the explanation does all the work for us and is quickly forgotten. If we look closely at the word "etymology," we see that it contains the word logos. The word *etymology* means the word of truth. Knowing a word's etymology provides us with a firm ground on which to stand. I could never understand why we decided to turn away from teaching etymology. If we are to have meaning within our lives, I think that the first place to turn is the meaning of words.

6 Janet Farrell Leontiou, *Communicating with Integrity* (Boston: Pearson Learning Solutions, 2013).

As was mentioned within the previous chapter, the word logos has many meanings and if we return to the Greek, so much of it is dependent upon the context in which it is used. The word logos means the word but not the word as we think of it. The word *logos* means the word as an ancient would see it. *Logos* means not only the word but everything behind the word: the meaning, the intention, the breath, the story, the history, and the study of. As previously stated, my students read a short essay called "Speaking the Corn Into Being" by the Native American writer Diane Glancy. The essay is not even two pages long, but it will take me months to teach the ideas contained within those pages. The author is writing from a cultural point of view, a similar culture to the ancient Greek, that is no longer our own.

The way in which Glancy is writing about the word might evoke the ancient concept of *logos*. For Glancy, and for me, the word is generative. We create worlds with our words. Glancy states that the Native American understood the god-like power in our capacity to speak. Glancy tells us that the Native American understood the power to create with words. This understanding resulted in the tremendous reverence the culture held toward spoken word. I take these teachings to heart when I teach that communication is holy work. I come to this conclusion by listening to the etymologies of the words connected with communication. The word "communication" itself means one together and it is etymologically connected to the word communion. The word respond means to pour liquids to the gods. The word symbol used to refer to a physical object that was broken in half and shared between guest and host. Should guest and host part ways and come together again, they may reunite the two halves and remember the hospitality once shared. If we remember this etymology for the word symbol, it leads us to a very different place than the denotation of symbol as representation. Glancy reminds us: "The breath forming words is holy."[7] I tell my students that if we remembered this each time we opened our mouths to speak, we would reduce the damage we do with our words. The psychologist James Hillman wrote of this same understanding

7 Glancy, "Speaking the Corn Into Being," *The Utne Reader*, September 1, 1997. https://www.utne.com/mind-and-body/speaking-the-corn-into-being-cherokee-oral-tradition

when he reminded us of the holy nature of communication: "We need to recall the angel aspect of the word, recognizing the words as independent carriers of soul between people."[8]

This view sees words, contrary to being nothing, as living beings. Words have ancestry and legacy. They come from somewhere, the etymology, and have a life. Words also have a legacy. Once I speak the words, I offer them to another and if the other remembers my words, they now (for better or worse) live inside another. My words are my legacy. This idea of memory, I think, is another aspect of spoken word that makes us stop and think before we speak. When I speak, I may become part of another if he or she remembers. Understanding this, leads me to ask the question: how is it that I wish to be remembered?

One of the first exercises I ask that my students engage in when they come into the class is to speak the story of their name. Some students are raised knowing their story and some have no idea. My intention is to shift them away from the view that their name is nothing special and merely something arbitrarily assigned. My wish is that they begin to change their attitude toward all words by first shifting their attitudes toward their names. The story of their names serves as a wonderful heuristic device to discover all that I wish for them to learn. In the concentration camps, the tatoo on the prisoners' arms replaced their names and solidified the prisoner being seen as number instead of a human being.

To set Frankl's book within the context of the power of spoken word is to understand that he, as a Jew, is living a life spoken into being by Hitler. Hitler used the word "parasite" to speak a reality into existence that the Jews were not human beings. This was an essential component in seeing what was done to the Jews was of no consequence. Hitler constructed the concentration camps through words before the physical barracks were constructed. The dehumanizing language of parasites planted the seeds that they needed to be removed and done away with in order to have a healthy Germany. Words are extremely economical—an entire world is within one word.

Within the context of the language of "parasite" I would say that every time we use dehumanizing language to refer to people, we are

8 James Hillman, *Re-Visioning Psychology* (New York: Harper & Row, 1975), 7.

on a very slippery slope. For instance, when a group of people are spoken about as "animals" (as we sometimes hear now) is to construct a group who are not people. If they are less than human, it does not much matter what we do with them or to them. This is an obvious example of the kind of power words have but many are not outraged by people being spoken of as animals. Now, let's take another more ubiquitous example of referring to the people who were murdered as the "extermination of the Jews." Each time I hear those words, I bristle. I do not think that those are the best of words. The word extermination means driven out, but I cannot remove the connotations of insects and/or bugs from the word "extermination." In the preface to one of the editions to *Man's Search for Meaning,* Gordon W. Allport writes: "How could he—every possession lost, every value destroyed, suffering from hunger, cold and brutality, hourly expecting extermination … ."[9] I would use the word death here instead of extermination. And for speaking about the Holocaust, I prefer the language of killing, murder and/or genocide.

All my academic degrees are in a subject—rhetoric—which is no longer part of the academic curriculum. Rhetoric was once part of the cornerstone of what was considered to be an educated person, but it has moved out of fashion. I do not think the decision to move away from the teaching of rhetoric was a good decision for us, but it went the way of Latin, Greek, and etymology. I say this because this pedagogical choice to exclude this subject has really left us in the dark. Rhetoric is synonymous with the word persuasion. As you will see throughout the pages of this book is that I see all words as persuasive so that persuasion is not a particular type of speech but is, in fact, the nature of speech.

It is often a habit to belittle spoken word and highlight its inferiority. Even Frankl does this twice within the book. Once when he is discussing how it is we who are questioned by life instead of doing the questioning, he states: "Our answer must consist, not in talk and meditation, but in right action and right conduct."[10] I do not think that this distinction helps us and instead I offer that speech is action—symbolic

9 Gordon W. Allport preface in Viktor E. Frankl, *Man's Search for Meaning* (New York: Simon & Schuster, 1959), 9–10.
10 Frankl, 77.

action and it is more productive to think of it as such. The second example is most baffling to me. Frankl is speaking about life within the camp and tells us: "The right example was more effective than words could ever be."[11] And then, "The immediate influence of behavior is always more effective than that of words."[12] Immediately following these words within the book, Frankl offers a beautiful example of the power of words. He is addressing behavior, but he is also suggesting the power in the labeling of the behavior. It is a long passage within the book and merits quoting in its entirety:

> It had been a long day. On parade, an announcement had been made about the many actions that would, from then on, be regarded as sabotage and therefore punishable by immediate death by hanging. Among these were crimes such as cutting small strips from our old blankets (in order to improvise ankle supports) and very minor "thefts." A few days previously a semi-starved prisoner had broken into the potato store to steal a few pounds of potatoes. The theft had been discovered and some prisoners had recognized the "burglar." When the camp authorities heard about it they ordered that the guilty man be given up to them or the whole camp would starve for a day. Naturally the 2,500 men preferred to fast.[13]

In this passage, Frankl is describing the behavior of solidarity but he is also using language to create a reality. The switch of words from starving to fasting points to the power of words. The switch brings with it the understanding that even within the camps, there was the element of choice. The word *starving* suggests that someone is prohibiting the ability to eat but *fasting* suggests that not eating is chosen for the higher good. Fasting also brings with it religious overtones that underscore Frankl's meaning.

The example offered above is one of many where Frankl is showing the tremendous power of spoken word while, at times, diminishing that power. The example noted serves as a case study in language. In every situation, there is a reality that is constant and unchanging (in this example, it is the scarcity of food) but what I call that scarcity is a

11 Frankl, 80.
12 Frankl, 80.
13 Frankl, 80–81.

choice. I look upon the words as frames that we construct that instruct us how to look upon reality.

There is an energy spectrum present within the frames—either positive, neutral, or positive. Fasting, here, obviously represents positive energy while starving suggests negativity.

One question to always ask about one's words or another person's words is: what kind of energetic charge the word has because that will tell you something about both the intention and how the word is received.

Frankl clearly was a gifted communicator and a gifted psychiatrist. Throughout the book, he tells several stories that I would place under the heading of shifting points of view. The power we possess is looking at one experience through several different lenses. Sometimes, we need help in doing this for ourselves and we require the help of others to generate different lenses. I think that the expression: "I never looked at it in that way" can, quite literally, save lives. Before providing a helpful word to another, we first need to understand how the other sees.

One common theme about effective communication from Aristotle up to present time is that our communication must be other centered. Our words need to be not for ourselves but for others. This becomes, in fact, a litmus test for our talk. We need to ask if the words we are about to speak are ultimately for ourselves or for the other? This other-centeredness is consistent with Frankl's call for us to be outwardly directed. Frankl's outward gaze is focused on how to best serve not so much ourselves but, instead, serve the world. In several places within the book, Frankl was able to offer words that removed a burden that the individual was carrying. One example was a discussion with a rabbi who was distraught because he had lost his entire family in the Holocaust and now, his current wife was sterile. At the core of his grief was the belief that he was eternally separated from his children because they died as innocent martyrs and he would die an old, sinful man. Frankl asks him: "Is it not conceivable, Rabbi, that precisely this was the meaning of your surviving your children: that you may be purified through these years of suffering, so that finally you, too, though not innocent like your children, may become worthy of joining them in Heaven?"[14]

14 Frankl, 120.

The rabbi was said to leave the encounter relieved of the suffering he had been carrying. Frankl introduces this other-centered message regarding communication when he states: "However, when a patient stands on the firm ground of religious belief, there can be no objection to making use of the therapeutic effect of his religious convictions and thereby drawing upon his spiritual resources."[15] Here, Frankl and the rabbi share the common ground of Judaism but it doesn't really matter if Frankl is devout or not because what matters is that the rabbi is devout.

Throughout the book, Frankl is offering examples from conversations taking place within a therapeutic setting but that does not mean that those conversations are only found within a professional setting. The examples are showing the kind of communication that occurs with people that are therapeutic (from the Greek, therapia, meaning to attend) and therefore may be lifesaving. He tells the story of a distraught physician who is drowning in grief after the loss of his wife. Frankl tells us:

> Now, how could I help him? What should I tell him? Well, I refrained from telling him anything but instead confronted him with the question "What would have happened, Doctor, if you had died first, and your wife would have to survive you?" "Oh," he said "for her this would have been terrible; how she would have suffered!" Whereupon I replied, "You see, Doctor, such a suffering has been spared her, and it was you who have spared her this suffering—to be sure, at the price that you now have to survive and mourn her."[16]

Frankl's story that he shared instructs us that instead of telling another how he or she is to feel, we should ask a question instead of making a pronouncement. If we follow the thinking of the ancients, wisdom is usually found within the question and not in the answer. Here, Frankl asks the doctor to imagine if things had gone differently and that question triggers the doctor to feel gratitude that he is the one left behind to mourn. Frankl concludes the story with: "In some way, suffering ceases to be suffering at the moment it finds a meaning such as the meaning of a sacrifice."[17] This comment provides us with some insight

15 Frankl, 119.
16 Frankl, 112–113.
17 Frankl, 113.

on how Frankl is instructing us to look upon sacrifice as a manifestation of being outwardly oriented. The example highlights the power in offering an alternate frame for the other. The creation of an alternative frame is more likely accomplished within the context of conversation than something that can be achieved while sitting in solitude. If we can open an alternate frame for another, it is nothing short of potentially saving someone's life.

Another powerful example of the shifting frames of language is when Frankl tells the story of a diplomat who came to see him for psychological counsel. He tells us that the man had been in therapy for five years and the narrative that the former psychologist offered was that the man did not like his job because he had unexamined authority issues that never were sorted out and that man needed to reconcile with his father. This example, to me, demonstrates a cautionary tale of how we can become persuaded into believing a reality that is not our own by someone who has authority. It is difficult to know, at times, who knows better—the other or myself? The answer depends on the situation. Sometimes I know best and sometimes the other knows best and I need to develop the discernment to know the difference. When we say blanket statements such as: "I always know what is best" is equally absurd as saying: "The other always knows best." What I need to remember always is that I need to respond and if I am acting as I have always acted, it is a reaction and not a response. From reading Frankl, we also know that every situation calls for a different response and that means that we always need to keep thinking. There is a quote attributed to Frankl:

> Between stimulus and response there is a space. In that space lies our freedom to choose our response. In our response lies our growth and freedom.[18]

I think that we sometimes forget to be mindful of the space between what someone says to us and how we choose to respond. We are

18 This quote is often attributed to Frankl however I cannot find it. While it may not be his exact language, it does follow Frankl's thinking as he has outlined it within the book.

oftentimes too quick to accept another's interpretation, and, at the same time, we are sometimes too quick to reject the other's interpretation.

In the example above, the former psychologist sounded Freudian and therefore he/she was looking at the analysand through a Freudian frame and saw the issue as relating to the patient's father. Frankl's insight was that the man in analysis was not really a patient and should not have been treated as such. The person was dissatisfied with his life because he was not doing his work. The man had been in therapy for five years and was being asked to accept a narrative that was not his own. Frankl told him that once he had embarked upon a change of professions, the issue was resolved.

Inspired by Frankl (who was himself inspired by the Stoics), I created my own theory of logostherapy—which means to attend to the word. I try to invite my students to see what the word is telling them by learning its etymology. Next, I invite them to listen to themselves. I know that this may sound trite but sometimes we are too close to listen to what we are saying. For example, I had a student write a paper about her own suicidal ideation when she was younger. At the beginning of the paper, she wrote about how much she hated that she had to pay attention to what others thought. At the end of the page she said that when she was in middle school, she wanted to take her own life but she then thought about what that act would do to her mother. Here, she is not listening to herself because she does not hear the contradiction. First, it is her choice whether she pays attention to what others think. Second, it was worrying what others would think that saved her life.

The last part of the trilogy of logostherapy is listening to what others say. In every situation, I need to remind myself that the words spoken by other people are their choice on how to construct a world. It need not be my choice. For example, after a particularly rough school year for my son with disability, my school district referred to my son as "medically fragile." This was because my son often missed school that year. He often missed school because the children in his class were sent to school even when very sick, their classroom was very small and there were no windows in their makeshift room. The environment was a perfect storm for breeding illnesses. It had gotten so bad that I asked his aide to call me if someone was ill within the class and we would come to take him home. My son has disability, but he is not medically fragile. It was the environment of the classroom, in my opinion, that needed remediation. It is, however, easier to construct the issue around my son instead of addressing the inadequacy of the physical plant to meet the needs of these children. I am not medically fragile, and I know that had I been placed in that environment, I would have gotten sick. The language of medically fragility is usually language offered by a healthcare professional. I also need to say that there was no bad intention in speaking these words. The words were offered with deep compassion but nevertheless, they were not true. I attempted to offer different words to describe the situation of my son's school experience that year. I attempted to shift those with whom I was speaking to focus on the environment as the issue instead of my son.

The three examples offered from Frankl were his attempts to do the same for his patients—to shift the patients' mindset to new places. The stories address the components of Frankl's three-part system for creating a meaningful life: love, work, and suffering. Two of the men were grieving the loss of their loves and needed a fresh way of seeing the suffering. The diplomat needed a new way of seeing his work. In the next chapter, I will merge my theory of logostherapy to Frankl's theory of logotherapy. By situating the words of the three parts of logotherapy within their etymologies, I think a stronger idea comes through regarding the place that love, work, and suffering has within our lives.

References

Cron, Lisa. *Wired for Story.* Berkeley, CA.: Ten Speed Press, 2012.

Culkin, John. "A Schoolman's Guide to Marshall McLuhan," *Saturday Review.* 18 March 1967, 70.

Farrell Leontiou, Janet. *Communicating with Integrity.* Boston, MA: Pearson Learning Solutions, 2013.

Glancy, Diane. "Speaking the Corn into Being," in *The West Pole.* Minneapolis: University of Minnesota Press, 1997. Also, *Utne Reader, 1* September 1997. https://utne.com/mind-and-body/speaking-the-corn-into-being-cherokee-oral-tradition

Hillman, James. *Re-Visioning Psychology.* New York: Harper & Row, 1975.

Jabr, Ferris. "The Reading Brain in the Digital Age: The Science of Paper Versus Screens," *Scientific America.* https://www.scientificamerican.com/article/reading-paper-screens/

Plato, *Phaedrus in Plato: Complete Works.* J.M. Cooper (ed.). Indianapolis, IN: Hackett, 1997.

Chapter Three

Logotherapy

The takeaway from Frankl's book is that if our lives have little meaning, it is because we have not put the meaning into our lives. This is not an accusation but instead, is a borrowing from the existential philosophy that runs throughout his work. Sometimes, we do act as if life comes to us with a pre-established meaning. To see our lives as meaningless is a starting place and an opportunity—not an ending place. Once we have the awareness, we can begin the work of constructing a meaningful life.

Frankl provides us with a blueprint on how to construct a meaningful life. Logotherapy, he tells us, consists of work, love, and suffering. In order to have a meaningful life, we must have these three parts. In this part of the book, I will look at the three words Frankl's offers (work, love, and suffering) and discuss how returning to the etymology of each word allows us to go deeper into what Frankl meant and begin to see how these three areas start to take shape within our own lives. In other words, here I will be merging Frankl's theory of logotherapy to my theory of logostherapy.

Let's begin with work. The word *work* comes from the Latin *opus* meaning one's grand purpose. The important distinction here is that our work is not our job. A job is a piece of a larger enterprise; it is something we do to pay bills and eat but our jobs have nothing to do with our purpose. This distinction is an important one. We should, in my opinion, begin to ask children how they envision their purpose/work when they are young, all the while understanding that their answer will shift as they age. When I talk to my students about this distinction, it is the first time they have heard it. I also tell them that at their age, they are not supposed to know what their work is, but they are supposed to be engaged with discovering what their work may be.

An important distinction here to make is that the difference between whether something is work or a job lies in the person and not in the activity. It is not true that janitorial work is a job while becoming a doctor is work. For some individuals, doctoring is a job and being a janitor is work. Some years ago, I was an AVP at Chase within their Investment Banking Division. After four years and four promotions, I knew that I needed to leave because it was not my work. I decided to return to school for my Ph.D. and then, teach full-time. While at Chase, I encountered many individuals for whom Investment Banking was their work. I knew it was not mine.

Sometimes if our work is something that we cannot make money doing, we will need to get jobs throughout our lives, to support our work. It will be a sacrifice, to be sure, and it is one that we need to go into with our eyes wide open. My former student, Michael (who became the illustrator for one of my books)[1] has known that he is a filmmaker since the age of 5. He does not yet make money through his films but instead needs to hold various jobs so that he can live and have the money to make his films. Michael, though, has never seen himself as anything but a filmmaker because that is his work. As I have stated, I came to realize my work later in life. All of us are on different paths and we need to honor the path that we each are on. It is easier if you know early what your work is because then, you can start to prepare yourself for doing your work.

1 Janet Farrell Leontiou, *The Doctor Still Knows Best: How Medical Culture is Still Marked by Paternalism* (New York: Peter Lang, 2020). Cartoons by Michael Staffieri, Jr.

Another feature of our work is that it changes as we do. I had a former student who was a lawyer when I met her. She had gone through the horrific experience of watching her husband die and leaving her with two young daughters to raise. The experience changed how she saw her work and she returned to school to become a nurse. When asked about why she was turning her life upside down to start over, her reply (as she reported in class) was: "Because I can." Her life. Her choice. Speaking her truth can inspire others to think they can too.

Sometimes our work shifts as does the circumstances of our lives. So much of my classroom teaching has turned to how we speak about the disabled; my work has shifted since I am raising a child with disabilities. Another aspect of work that has shifted since having my son, is that I have written two books on medical communication because, again, that is where my life has taken me. When seen through the lens of Stoicism I am given certain conditions within my life and in giving these conditions meaning, I am making sense of my own experience and hopefully, in writing my books, helping others to make sense of their own experience as well. I am making the point that if we struggle to create meaning, it serves not only ourselves but also serves others who can see themselves through another.

When we begin to engage with the nature of our work, we see that it is much bigger than a way to make money. We most commonly equate money with success, and I would like to now address what Frankl tells us about success:

> Don't aim at success-the more you aim at it and make it a target, the more you are going to miss it. For success, like happiness, cannot be pursued; it must ensue, and it only does so as the unintended side-effect of one's dedication to a cause greater than oneself or as the by-product of one's surrender to a person other than oneself. Happiness must happen, and the same holds for success: you have to let it happen by not caring about it.[2]

This quote comes in the preface by Frankl and leaves us with much to unpack. First, is the radical quality of the statement: do not aim at success. This is truly counter-cultural to all that we have been taught

2 Frankl, xiv–xv.

within this goal driven and bottom-line focused culture. He is not telling us to take the steps required to reach a goal but instead is telling us to forget the end result entirely. He is telling us that we have a better shot at reaching the goal when we forget about the goal. The language I offer to help my students make sense of the quote is process versus product.

Process means that we engage for engagement's sake and forget about where it is going. Product means that we come into the experience focused on getting out or what we may get out of it. These are two different approaches to life, and they pertain to everything we do: jobs, school, sports, relationships, etc. Once we focus on the end of something, we kill meaning and the more we commit ourselves to engaging with the experience, the more likely we end up successful. Take the example of the classroom. The student who comes into the class focused on getting an A is less likely to end up with that grade because the student is focused on the end result instead of engaging with learning the material for its own sake. For the latter student, the grade is a byproduct for having learned the material well.

After twenty-seven years of teaching within a community college, I think that my students are more ill- prepared for college with each passing year. I am not saying that they are less intelligent, but I am noticing a lack of preparation. I realize that the causation for this is complicated but the greater emphasis we place on the future and chasing after the product, the less I see that my students are capable of succeeding in anything. It seems to me that we have exchanged meaning with a promise of greater achievement in the future and under this model, I fear that my students will have nothing.

Frankl uses the word *ensue* and not the word *pursue.* He is telling us to stop chasing after something and instead, to trust that if we do our work, success will come to us. He is not, however, telling us (as my students sometimes think) that success will find you when you are doing nothing. His choice of words is quite strong. He tells us to dedicate ourselves to a cause greater than ourselves. The word *dedicate* has Latin roots and it means to consecrate to a deity or a cause greater than ourselves—our work. He is telling us to look upon our work as holy and to give everything we have to it. If we do that, success is the byproduct of the choice to live this way.

I encourage my students to develop the metanoia of engaging with the process instead of aiming at the product. When I ask that they engage with the process, I am asking that my students think for the sake of thinking. Not thinking to get to a specific place but instead to think and go to wherever their thoughts take them. My students come to me having been indoctrinated within a system that trains them in attaining closure and getting to the correct answer. I agree with the thinker, Hannah Arendt, who speaks of closure as the end of thought.[3] I attempt to speak to my students about those times when we thought that we did get to the correct answer, only to learn that we were wrong.

I offer my students the language of process versus product to provide them with a way of thinking about everything. Frankl is offering a process-oriented way to think about success, but the framework is relevant to every aspect of life. That is why I call for a metanoia. I ask my students to reflect on how it is they come into an experience, significantly shapes that experience. We live within a culture that is almost exclusively product driven.

Let's return to how Frankl speaks of success. The other way to become successful, according to Frankl, is to surrender to someone other than oneself. In other words, we become successful by dedicating our lives to work and/or surrendering our lives to love. He chooses the word surrender here to suggest a complete giving in to love without reservation. If we live our lives as Frankl states here, success will become the unintended consequence of a life well-lived with meaning.

If I may return to the radicalness of Frankl's statement about success because I think that, at times, readers overlook the nuance here. Within our culture, the only value that we seem to possess is the value of money and here Frankl tells us: "people have enough to live by but nothing to live for; they have the means but no meaning."[4] Students tell me that what it is they want out of life is to make a lot of money. I try to

3 Hannah Arendt, *Men in Dark Times* (New York: Harcourt Brace Jovanovich, 1971), 8–10.

4 Frankl, 140.

invite them to hear just how absurd that sounds (even if it is common). People mostly do not make money because they want to make money but instead make money because they have discovered their work, are good at it, and people are willing to pay them to do it. We tend, within the culture, to worship business leaders who make lots of money and we want what they have. We cannot have what they have because they have discovered their work and we must do the same. We cannot take someone else's work and graft it on to our lives because it will not work. We have seen many start-ups get sold for a very handsome sum. The entrepreneur does not usually retire but instead usually starts another company because being an entrepreneur is the person's work. The same goes for the athletes whom the culture worships. The reason why the athlete makes so much money is because, for him or her, that sport is his/her work.

The next leg of logotherapy is love. Love, as Frank, tells us is our highest purpose.[5] I think that in order to grasp Frankl's meaning, it is helpful to understand that in the Greek language there are several different words for expressing different types of love. I think that Frankl is talking about something bigger than our own personal relationships here. Our relationships are part of our response, but the concept is much deeper. I think of the Greek word agape, meaning all-giving and unconditional love expressed toward our fellow human beings. Agape is sometimes referred to as love in action and it signifies a way of being in the world.

Frankl, throughout the book, is tapping into the wisdom found within every faith tradition that we should be outwardly focused on what it is we can give. For instance, when Frankl speaks of attitude, this is precisely what he means. Let's look at two examples of how he uses the word attitude and the context for each:

> We who lived in concentration camps can remember the men who walked through the huts comforting others, giving away their last piece of bread. They may have been few in number, but they offer sufficient proof that everything can be taken from men but one thing: the last of human freedoms—to

5 Frankl, 37.

> choose one's attitude in any given set of circumstances, to choose one own way.[6]

This example is striking, of course, because the giving occurred within a situation where people were starving. I cannot imagine the capacity to give within a context where the need for self-preservation was so great.

The next place within the book where Frankl speaks about attitude expands upon the connection that giving is the point of living:

> What was really needed was a fundamental change in our attitude toward life. We had to learn ourselves and, furthermore, we had to teach the despairing men, that it really did not matter what we expected from life, but rather what life expected from us.[7]

This is an important shift Frankl is making in this passage. Instead of looking at what we can get, instead ask what we can give. Frankl is also tapping into the Stoic mentality that the world does not care about our expectations. Life is not here to satisfy our expectations and in fact, our expectations frequently get in the way. Frankl is subscribing to the point of view that the world owes us nothing but instead it is we who owe the world.

The entire discussion of giving versus getting, at first, sounds counterintuitive. The more I focus on getting, the less I receive. Frankl is living in accordance with every faith tradition that states when one gives with a pure heart and expects nothing in return, that is when one receives. Through personal experience, I know that this is correct. One example that comes to mind is attending church service within my spouse's religion as a gift to him. I decided to leave my church after I was graduated from catholic school. My choice to enter a Greek Orthodox church one Palm Sunday morning as a gift to my spouse led me to meet a priest who changed my life. I ended up studying orthodoxy with this man and at the culmination of the studies, I decided to convert. I never

6 Frankl, 65–66.
7 Frankl, 77.

expected anything like that to happen for me in making the choice to attend church.[8]

When looked at within this context, this may be the thinking behind those well-intentioned suggestions that when facing depression, it may be helpful to volunteer and serve others. Of course, I am not here suggesting that a person is able to volunteer to help others when faced with debilitating depression. It is cruel, indeed, to tell someone to just get on with it when he or she can barely get out of bed. What this suggestion does speak to is that we may be able to shake off our own blues by giving to others because what we end up receiving back takes us to a new place.

Frankl's discussion of self-actualization is addressed within the context of love. It should be noted that the language of self-actualization comes from the American psychologist, Abraham Maslow. Frankl and Maslow were contemporaries. Both were writing about humans at his/her best. Frankl states that we reach our greatest potential as human beings when we give to others. Frankl, when asked during a lecture how an individual may discover one's purpose, answered the question in this way: "The meaning of your life is to help others find the meaning of theirs."[9] Let's look at some additional words of Frankl's on the matter:

> By declaring that man is responsible and must actualize the potential meaning of his life, I wish to stress that the true meaning of life is to be discovered in the world rather than within man or his own psyche, as though it were a closed system. I have termed this constitutive characteristic "the self-transcendence of human existence." It denotes the fact that being human always points, and is directed, to something, or someone, other than oneself—be it a meaning to fulfill or another human being to encounter. The more one forgets himself—by giving himself to a cause to serve or another person to love—the more human he is and the more he actualizes himself.[10]

8 See Janet Farrell Leontiou, "The Convergence," *The Hellenic Chronicle*, Vol. LXXXVIII No. 6, 11 August 1999, Part 1, p. 1; Vol. LXXXVIII No. 7, 18 August 1999, Part 2, p. 5; Vol. LXXXVIII No. 8, 25 August 1999, Part 3, p. 4; LXXXVIII No. 9, 1 Sept. 1999, Part 4, p. 10.

9 As quoted by William J. Winslade in Afterword to Viktor E. Frankl, *Man's Search for Meaning* (Boston: Beacon Press, 2006), 165.

10 Frankl, 110–111.

This idea that Frankl is developing here connects us back with his discussion about success. Our work must be directed toward the world and not be directed toward the self. The discussion connects us back to the point I made about process versus product. Within this context, Frankl addresses the fact that we never reach self-actualization because we are an ongoing work in progress. We are never done, and we are never finished. Frankl offers a cautionary note that, like success, we cannot aim for it:

> What is called self-actualization is not attainable at all, for the simple reason that the more one would strive for it, the more he would miss it. In other words, self-actualization is possible only as a side-effect of self-transcendence.[11]

Frankl speaks about challenging others to tap into their potential as an act of love. I love his discussion of seeing potential within another or in other words, in seeing what is not yet present. He tells us that it is through love, agape, that we can begin to see the potential within another and thereby help the other to see it too. I cannot help but to think of my own situation and my work in raising a son who has disabilities. I have always worked to have him surrounded by those who see potential in him. Some people, instead, see the hardware of a wheelchair and that is all they see. One year, I gifted all those who work with my son with a framed quote by the philosopher, Martin Heidegger: "Higher than actuality stands *possibility*."[12] I love that quote because it asks me to look for and to see the possible within others, within the moment, and within myself.

I carry another quote with me to serve as a reminder and this one comes from the writer Goethe: "If we treat people as they are, we make them worse but if we treat people as if they were what they ought to be, we help them become what they are capable of becoming."[13] When my son began school, I witnessed the kids embody Goethe's sentiment.

11 Frankl, 111.

12 Heidegger, *Being and Time*. Tans. John Macquarrie & Edward Robinson (New York: Harper & Row, 1962), 63.

13 From a search, this quote is from Johann Wolfgang von Goethe, *Wilhelm Meister's Apprenticeship*, Book 8, Chapter 4.

I wished for his classmates to see him as so much more than an extension of a wheelchair. I showed the children a slide show of my son doing—walking, riding his bike, swimming with dolphins, parasailing, skiing, etc. All of these activities needed to be adapted, of course, but I wished for these very small children to see that he can do things in the world and just maybe, he may have done even more than they did in their very young lives. My presentation had some amazing effects on the kids. One child, whose mother I know, said: "Did you know that Andreas can walk? If he can, that means that we can help him." This boy's comments go to the heart, I think, of what Frankl, Heidegger, and Goethe were saying. He, at the tender age of 5, understands.

Frankl tells us that there are two races: the decent and indecent.[14] He tells us that there is no predetermined thinking present in determining who belongs to each category. People are either decent or indecent depending upon one's actions and words. He tells us that each is found in all groups of society: "In this sense, no group is of 'pure race'—and therefore one occasionally found a decent fellow among the camp guards."[15] It is interesting to note that this comment is the closest Frankl comes to speaking about Hitler within this book and even here, remains unnamed. The person who attempted to eliminate all Jews, has instead been removed from these pages.

Frankl is taking the important step here in claiming that not all the prisoners were angels, and not all the guards were devils. Life is always much more complicated than that. You cannot tell the heroes from the villains by the uniform. He tells us that the Capos, fellow Jews, were more brutal than the German guards and we know from Holocaust narratives,[16] that some prisons made it out alive because of the actions taken by a guard. Sometimes the foreman was kind:

14 Frankl, 86.

15 Frankl, 86.

16 See Roman Polanski's 2002 film "The Pianist" which tells the true story of one concentration camp prisoner who was aided by a Nazi and this aide, combined with his music, led to his survival. The film is an adaptation from the book by Wladyslaw Szpilman, *The Pianist: The Extraordinary True Story of One Man's Survival in Warsaw, 1939–1945* (New York: Picador, 1946).

> I remember how one day a foreman secretly gave me a piece of bread which I knew he must have saved from his breakfast ration. It was far more than the small piece of bread which moved me to tears at that time. It was the human "something" which this man also gave to me—the word and look which accompanied the gift.[17]

The human something Frankl is speaking of is the acknowledgement of being seen as a human being. I know that in circumstances not even remotely parallel, within a school for instance, students will sometimes be treated like their identification number and not as human beings. I have seen, too, the relief come in the form of tears, to finally be acknowledged as a fellow human being.

When speaking to my students about this attitude that Frankl argues is the preferred way to be within the world, I tell my students that the care we extend to each other is the mark of whether we live within a civilized culture or uncivilized one. One of my students asked me for the evidence of my claim. My mind went to the anthropologist Margaret Mead's response to what she considered the first sign of civilization in a culture:

> Mead said that the first sign of civilization in an ancient culture was a femur (thighbone) that had been broken and then healed. Mead explained that in the animal kingdom, if you break a leg, you die. You cannot run from danger, get to the river for a drink or hunt for food. You are meat for prowling beasts. No animal survives a broken leg long enough for the bone to heal. A broken femur that has healed is evidence that someone has taken time to stay with the one who fell, has bound up the wound, has carried the person to safety and has tended the person through recovery. Helping someone else through difficulty is where civilization starts.[18]

Frankl speaks of human potential at its best as transforming a personal tragedy into a triumph.[19] In another chapter, I will write about how this language invokes the Nietzschean ideal of the uberman but for now, it is the beginning of Frankl's final way of how we may create meaning

17 Frankl, 86.
18 As found in Ira Byock, *The Best Care Possible: A Physician's Quest to Transform Care Through the End of Life* (New York: Avery Publishing, 2012).
19 Frankl, 112.

within our lives. The third part of logotherapy is suffering. Frankl tells us we create meaning by making sense of unavoidable suffering. His language is very clear—if we can avoid it, we should avoid it but if it is unavoidable, it must be for some purpose.

Frankl is again relying on the ancient Stoics for guidance who believed that suffering is the human condition. A Stoic response to "why me" would be "why not me?" Our usual understanding of the stoic as someone who does not display his or her emotions may be instructive here. According to ancient Stoic philosophy, everything is perceived as a gift from the gods so therefore, everything (including the suffering) is for our own good. We would never choose to suffer but as the Stoics understood, humans need to have the judgment to understand that which they can control and that which is outside the realm of control. Without suffering and death, Frankl tells us life cannot be complete: "If there is meaning in life at all, then there must be a meaning in suffering. Suffering is an ineradicable part of life, even as fate and death."[20]

To fully appreciate Frankl's meaning of suffering, I will once again turn to the Greek language. The word that closely resembles what Frankl means by suffering is pathos. Pathos means emotion, feeling, or passion. Frankl tells us that it was Spinoza who said: "Emotion, which is suffering, ceases to be suffering as soon as we form a clear and precise picture of it."[21] Here, Frankl is providing us with the opportunity to see the gift-like quality in our suffering. When people speak of the passion of Jesus Christ, for instance, they are speaking about the crucifixion and the resurrection; they are speaking about Good Friday and Easter Sunday.

Frankl invokes the words of the author Dostoevsky: "There is only one thing that I dread: not to be worthy of my suffering."[22] Frankl states: "The way in which a man accepts his fate and the suffering it entails, the way in which he takes up his cross gives him ample

20 Frankl, 67.
21 Frankl, 74.
22 Frankl, 66.

opportunity—even under the most difficult circumstances—to add deeper meaning to his life."[23]

Each of us is called upon to see this deeper meaning and frequently it is the suffering that speaks the loudest to capture our attention. Anyone who has ever suffered will, I think, immediately resonate with the analogy that Frankl offers to speak about suffering:

> A man's suffering is similar to the behavior of gas. If a certain quantity of gas is pumped into an empty chamber, it will fill the chamber completely and evenly, no matter how big the chamber. Thus suffering completely fills the human soul and conscious mind, no matter whether the suffering is great or little. Therefore the "size" of human suffering is absolutely relative.[24]

In this passage, Frankl makes such an important point about suffering. Here are the takeaway points for me: (1) if a person perceives that she or he is suffering, she or he is. To acknowledge someone else's pain has nothing to do with whether I would perceive it as pain. This is especially true regarding children. We sometimes look at a child's pain through an adult lens and therefore miss the point. (2) I do not need to compare my pain to another's pain because it is not a competition. We sometimes see our suffering as so much greater and therefore dismiss another's pain. (3) We sometimes compete for the prize of who carries the greatest pain. This is a bizarre quality in humans when people compete for the title of who can be the most miserable.

Frankl offers two stories from his time as a psychiatrist that demonstrate how we can offer an alternate frame to a person who is suffering. Sometimes the construction of an alternate frame is too difficult for us to accomplish on our own and we need the words of another to accomplish it. Once we create an alternate frame, it may be the equivalent of throwing a drowning person a life-preserver. One example that I have written about previously, that bears repeating is the story that Frankl tells of his encounter with a rabbi. Frankl tells us that there is no reservation about using the other's religious convictions to draw upon spiritual resources and placing himself in the shoes of the rabbi.

23 Frankl, 67.
24 Frankl, 44.

Frankl is making use of the understanding that effective communication is other-centered and developing empathy is a way of making oneself useful within the conversation. The rabbi visited Frankl because of the profound grief he experienced at the loss of his first wife and six children in Auschwitz. His grief was compounded as his second wife was sterile and there was no potential of having a son who would pray for him upon his death. Frankl asked the rabbi the question if he expected to be reunited with his deceased children in Heaven? Then, with tears, came the reason for his profound loss and it had to do with the afterlife more than grief associated with the loss of one's children within this life. The rabbi felt that he was eternally separated from his children because they were innocent martyrs and would surely ascend to Heaven. He, as he perceived himself, was an old, sinful man and would be denied entry into the Kingdom of Heaven. Frankl said to him:

> Is it not conceivable, Rabbi, that precisely this was the meaning of your surviving your children: that you may be purified through years of suffering, so that you, too, though not innocent like your children, may *become* worthy of joining them in Heaven?[25]

This exchange highlights the potential of what we can do for each other and how we may be able to respond to someone who is suffering. The exchange requires: thought, time, patience, imagination, care, empathy, helpfulness, understanding, responsibility, and the capacity to ask good questions. I highlight this list to reinforce that effective communication is not a skill or a trick but the result of formulating a thoughtful response to a fellow human being. The effect of this conversation, though, is that the rabbi found relief from deep suffering by being offered a new frame.

Frankl tells the story of another patient who was suffering the loss of his beloved wife. Frankl asks what he could tell this man and then offers that he told him nothing but asked a question. Frankl reminds us that we cannot speak to any person if we do not understand him or her. I frequently ask my students to invoke the Socratic ideal and to attempt to think of the question instead of the pronouncement. The question

25 Frankl, 120.

Frankl asks is if the man could imagine if his wife had survived him? The man responded that he would have never wanted that because of imagining how his wife would have suffered. Frankl replied: "You see, Doctor, such a suffering has been spared her, and it was you who have spared her this suffering—to be sure, at the price that now you have to survive and mourn her."[26] Then, to his readers, Frankl states: "In some way, suffering ceases to be suffering at the moment it finds a meaning, such as the meaning of a sacrifice."[27]

I would like to conclude this chapter by reinforcing that to have a meaningful life, we must have work, love, and suffering. The most difficult part of this equation is to make room for the suffering. I would like to conclude this chapter with the words of Gordon W. Allport who wrote a preface for an earlier edition of Frankl's book. Allport is discussing the strategies outlined within the book for preserving the remnants of one's life although the chances for surviving are slight. He offers these words: "Hunger, humiliation, fear and deep anger at injustices are rendered tolerable by closely guarded images of beloved persons, by religion, by a grim sense of humor, and even by glimpses of the healing beauties of nature—a tree or a sunset."[28] I conclude with this passage because it is a reminder that life consists of both suffering and love. We need to see both because both are omnipresent. We need to remind ourselves that if we are just seeing the darkness, we are only seeing part of life. The light is also present but maybe we are missing it. Remember also that if you do not yet have the meaning for your suffering, there is only pain. You will need to get to the other side to see what meaning the suffering has given to you. Be patient. We only construct meaning in retrospect. Frankl is quoted with: "That which is to give light must endure burning."[29] Whatever one has suffered may be

26 Frankl, 113.

27 Frankl, 113.

28 Gordon W. Allport's preface in Viktor E. Frankl, *Man's Search for Meaning* (New York: Simon & Schuster, Inc., 1959), 11.

29 This quote is usually attributed to Frankl's *Man's Search for Meaning* but I have not been able to locate the quote within the book. The cover of the Beacon Press paperback edition of Frankl's *Man's Search for Meaning* consists of a back background and a single burning flame. Like all symbols, the image has many meanings—suffering, education, and memorialization.

useful in helping others find their way. Choosing to live life in this most unselfish way is, as Frankl tells us, the greatest expression of humanity.

References

Allport, Gordon. Preface in Viktor E. Frankl's *Man's Search for Meaning.* New York: Simon & Schuster, 1959.

Arendt, Hannah. *Men in Dark Times.* New York: Harcourt Brace Jovanovich, 1971.

Byock, Ira. *The Best Care Possible: A Physician's Quest to Transform Care Through the End of Life.* New York: Avery Publishing, 2012.

Farrell Leontiou, Janet. *The Doctor Still Knows Best: How Medical Culture is Still Marked by Paternalism.* New York: Peter Lang, 2019.

———. "The Convergence." *The Hellenic Chronicle,* Vol. LXXXVIII No. 6, 11 August 1999, Part 1. Vol. LXXXVIII No. 7, 18 August 1999, Part 2. LXXXVIII No 8, 25 August 1999, Part 3.

Frankl, Viktor E. *Man's Search for Meaning.* Boston: Beacon Press, 2006.

Goethe, Johann Wolfgang von. *Wilhelm Meister's Apprentice.* H.M. Waidson, trans. Kalamazoo, MI: River Run Press, 1982. Book 8.

Heidegger, Martin. *Being and Time.* John Macquarrie & Edward Robinson, trans. New York: Harper & Row, 1962.

Szpilman, Wladyslaw. *The Pianist: The Extraordinary True Story of One Man's Survival in Warsaw, 1939–1945.* New York: Avery Publishing, 2012.

Chapter Four

The Existential Vacuum

Sometimes when people feel lost within their lives, they blame themselves. People may see a lack of meaning within their lives as personal failure. This makes the burden carried even heavier. There is a passage within Frankl's book that describes how we arrived at our current condition, and it is worthwhile to address because within a short passage, he seems to explain so much. I will begin by offering the paragraph:

> The existential vacuum is a widespread phenomenon of the twentieth century. This is understandable; it may be due to a twofold loss which man has had to undergo since he became a truly human being. At the beginning of human history, man lost some of his basic animal instincts in which an animal's behavior is embedded and by which it is secured. Such security, like Paradise, is closed to man forever; man has to make choices. In addition to this, however, man has suffered another loss in his more recent development inasmuch as the traditions which buttressed his behavior are now rapidly diminishing. No instinct tells him what he has to do, and no tradition tells him what he ought to do; sometimes he does not even know what he wishes

> to do. Instead, he either wishes to do what other people do (conformism) or he does what people wish him to do (totalitarianism).[1]

Frankl is telling us that our gut reactions used to inform us. We knew that we were safe or should be fearful based upon information from our gut. I think that in many cases, we have turned away from our gut reactions. This is not to say that our guts are always right, but I think it is useful to give our gut reactions a hearing. For instance, children are sometimes picking up on information not noticed by adults. They may express a discomfort with the presence of a particular adult's company and especially if the adult is a relative, the child may be punished for saying something unkind about a family member. The child may be, however, reacting to something the child is experiencing. After we moved away from using instinct to guide our path, Frankl talks about how we have moved away from the traditions that used to inform our lives. Some traditions that Frankl may be talking about may be oral traditions, family or religion. The stories we used to tell (from mythology, The Bible, or literature) contained lessons on how one was to live one's life. In the past, the family that you were born into predicted the trajectory of your life. Religion, too, used to have much more of a hold on us in the past and it regulated daily life regarding practices and activities. Frankl is not romantically speaking about the past but merely stating a factual reality that life did not require as much personal choice in the past. We can look at insular religious communities like the Amish or the Orthodox Jewish communities to see an example of the traditions holding a similar level of pre-established meaning within people's lives. For better or worse, children who grow up within these communities know what is expected of them.

The next part of the quote, Frankl is stating that for most of us our lives are open to choice but rather than revel in the openness of the vast array of choices before us, we become overwhelmed by the choices and succumb to either copying what others do (conform) or obey by doing what others tell us to do (totalitarianism). I think that this is such an important point Frankl is making. When faced with the ability of

1 Frankl, 106.

choosing whatever we wish, we need to remember to see that the selection process is just that—part of the process and to remember that we are abundantly fortunate to have so many options. Instead, what usually happens (and I see this behavior within my students) is that we forfeit our own capacity to choose and become followers—either conform or obey. In this moment of conformity or obedience, we have abdicated our capacity to choose.

I think that we have a propensity to forget that we are free. I see it when students come to college and instead of seeing that they can study anything they choose, they follow and do what others do—liberal arts. Their language seems to be embedded with shame for not specializing because when asked what they are studying, the response is usually the same: "just liberal arts." I think, by the way, that following a liberal arts course of study at the community college level makes all the sense in the world. I would like to see it more actively chosen instead of a program taken by default.

Frankl ends the quote with the word "totalitarianism." This is the closest that the author comes to referencing Hitler within the book and he does so without using his name. I think that it is a most interesting rhetorical choice—to remove the name of the man who attempted to obliterate the Jewish population shall himself be unnamed.

Frankl then goes on to explain the mindset of those who experience the existential vacuum.

"The existential vacuum manifests itself mainly in a state of boredom."[2] What does it mean to say that you are bored? If we take the starting place that all communication is about oneself, what we are saying when we proclaim that something is boring is that we are boring. Everything has the potential to become interesting; interest is a choice.

Frankl quotes the philosopher Schopenhauer's observation that "mankind was apparently doomed to vacillate eternally between the two extremes of distress and boredom."[3]

In my experience, those who know the most are usually people who are not bored. The more vibrant the life of the mind is, the more

2 Frankl, 106.
3 Frankl, 106.

interested and interesting the person is. Without meaning, we merely react between the two extremes of feeling stressed or bored. As Frankl repeatedly states within the book, a meaningless life is not sustainable.

I think that schools, unknowingly and unintentionally, create an existential vacuum for students. They do this in several ways. (1) Stressing product over process as in the language spoken of earlier doing things not for their intrinsic worth but instead to "get them over with." (2) Instructing the students to focus on the future instead of attending to the present. They are often told, for instance, to take Advanced Placement classes not for what they will learn but because they look good on their transcript when applying for college. (3) Downplaying the world of school. Students are often told that school is "not the real world." I think that this language has negative consequences for the students. I will later link this language of "real world" to creating a sense of provisional existence for the students.

I wish that we would stop talking to young people in such a way that erodes meaning. It is not intentionally hurtful, but I think it is the result of school officials not thinking about what their words are doing. We see a fair share of young people who become lost and instead of trying to understand how they became lost, we blame them. This always strikes me as particularly unfair because if there is anyone to blame, it is the adults. There is no maliciousness involved but adults often erode meaning from young peoples' experiences. This is exactly what happened as I sat in my typically developing son's school auditorium as he completed the eighth grade. Our district has a volunteer requirement to be completed prior to graduation. The school official spoke to the kids: "In between eighth and ninth grade, you have lots of down time, so it is a good time to get your volunteer hours over with." This example is an especially wasted opportunity if we think of the thesis offered by Frankl that giving is the key to everything about life. It is the key to our purpose. It is the key to our greatest expression of humanity. Here, it became one more thing to tick off the list on the way to graduation. The consequences for this language erode meaning for the students and may have the consequence that the students do more damage than good in their role as volunteers.

Most of my students are the products of broken systems. For the most part, students who end up in a community college are not those students who have managed to excel and play the game of school as well as some of their peers. They are in school because they have been told that they need a diploma to be able to do anything in the world, but they come into school, not expecting much of it. For the sixteen weeks that I have them, it is up to me and Frankl to change their minds.

I also think that apathy plays a significant role within my students. I do not think that adults fully understand that when we push young people to accomplish goals to check things off a list, we are doing a great deal of damage. This mentality strips experience of meaning and creates apathy. As Frankl states, apathy may have its place when people are coping with trauma. He calls apathy the second stage of prisoner psychology that the prisoners experienced as a way to get through the horror that surrounded them. When he uses the language of stages, he is suggesting that it is not meant to be something permanent. This, I think, is the difference between apathy within the Jewish prisoner and apathy within my students. The apathy that I see within my students is the result of participating within a system that seems to have little or no intrinsic meaning. Like most situations, the students are responsible for their own apathy, but they are not to blame. It is, without a doubt, the adults who have created the meaninglessness and then blame the young people when they act out because of the lack of meaning. Of course, none of this is malicious. In fact, I can see how many adults think that this hyper focus on goals is for the young people's best interest. In the next chapter, I will address how this emphasis on the future is not the best choice.

References

Frankl, Viktor E. *Man's Search for Meaning.* Boston: Beacon Press, 2006.

Chapter Five

The Tenses

Within the previous chapters, I wrote about the effects of asking students to almost exclusively focus on the future. I wrote about how focusing on the product is future directed. I also spoke about how when we aim at the end and make everything a means to an end, we destroy the capacity to create meaning. Frankl speaks about how focusing on the future can helpful in creating meaning because one can look toward what one wishes to accomplish. One may look toward a future accomplishment but not at the expense of negating the present. I think that we need to live in all three tenses simultaneously—live in the present, remember the past and plan for the future. There is much written about living in the present as in the present moment is all we have but if we live exclusively in the moment, it could lead to impulsivity. There is the potential to get stuck in any one of the temporal states. Too much focus on the present can lead to lack of planning for a future. Too much focusing on the future may lead to lack of memory because we are never truly present within the moment. Too much focus on the past, leads to nostalgia.

Nostalgia, from the Greek meaning longing for home, is what Frankl witnessed within some of the prisoners who led a provisional existence:

> Regarding our "provisional existence" as unreal was in itself an important factor in causing the prisoner to lose their hold on life; everything in a way became pointless. Such people forgot that often it is such an exceptionally difficult external situation which gives man the opportunity to grow spiritually beyond himself. Instead of taking the camp's difficulties as a test of their inner strength, they did not take their lives seriously and despised it as of something of no consequence. They preferred to close their eyes and to live in the past. Life for such people became meaningless.[1]

The nostalgia that Frankl describes within this passage is an exclusive preoccupation with the past. I attempt to teach my students the tricky balance of honoring the past through an act of remembrance. Remembering is different from nostalgia in that the latter implies that the person is stuck in the past. For each class, I ask students to write a reflection. The reflections serve the same purpose as a diary. It is a way to use the writing to engage in thought and to construct meaning. I ask that the students begin each class by reading their reflections from the previous class. In doing this, I am asking that students begin to navigate this space where they take their experience seriously and they start to pull together the past, the present and the future. I am also asking that they initiate—start something. I understand how difficult it is to start—start to do the work, start to ask the questions, start a conversation—but nothing will happen unless we choose to start. Frankl recognizes that those in the camp who were living lives of provisional existence were fearful of "making decisions and of taking any sort of initiative whatsoever."[2]

To become nostalgic is a condition that occurs when we are not on good terms with the present. Regret is when we are not on good terms with the past. Frankl presents us the philosophy of Kant's categorical

1 Frankl, 72.
2 Frankl, 56.

imperative to stave off regret and it serves as another example where the three tenses conflate:

> "Live as if you were living already for the second time and as if you had acted the first time as wrongly as you are about to act now!" It seems to me that there is nothing which would stimulate a man's sense of responsibleness more than this maxim, which invites him to imagine first that the present is past and second, that the past may yet be changed and amended. Such a precept confronts him with life's finiteness as well as the finality of what he makes out of both his life and himself.[3]

Here, Frankl is telling us to think before we act or speak because what is done cannot be undone. Often, damage is done because of lack of thought and not because of a malicious intention. Practicing the categorical imperative is developing the discipline of mind to think about consequences of words and actions before they are spoken or taken.

As I am writing this book, we approaching our two-year anniversary of living through a pandemic. I hear people speak in much the same way that Frankl describes provisional existence. He describes those who thought of their experiences as unreal and then failed to rise to the challenge that the situation presented. He could be speaking of us when he states when we do not see the potential that the current moment presents.

Frankl not only speaks of seeing potential within the situation but to see potential within the other. Within his discussion of seeing the potential of the other, Frankl speaks of it as a tension: "Such a tension is inherent in the human being and therefore is indispensable to mental well-being. We should not, then, be hesitant about challenging man with a potential meaning for him to fulfill."[4] In other words, Frankl is writing about the tension arising between who one is and who one wishes to become. This discussion reminds me of the words of Goethe: "If we treat people as they are we make them worse but if we treat people as if they were what they ought to be, we help them become what they are capable of becoming."[5] I have always loved this quote because it stresses that

3 Frankl, 109.
4 Frankl, 105.
5 Goethe, *Wilhelm Meister's Apprentice,* Book 8, Ch. 4.

which is possible. These words have been most instructive in choosing people to aid my son. I need to choose people who can see potential beyond the hardware of a wheelchair. Frankl tells us that it is love (or agape) that permits us to see potential:

> By his love he is enabled to see the essential traits and features in the beloved person; and even more, he sees that which is potential in him, which is not yet actualized but yet ought to be actualized. Furthermore, by his love, the loving person enables the beloved person to actualize these potentialities.[6]

It is clear to me that Frankl is speaking about agape and not just eros. The teacher, then, through agape may see the potential within the student and help the student to strive to actualize his or her potential. Frankl also tells us that self-actualization is not attainable. If we recall the earlier Frankl quote offered about success. If we strive for it, the more we miss it. "In other words," Frankl tells us, "self-actualization is possible only as a side-effect of self-transcendence."[7] In keeping with the attitude that Frankl offers as the preferred way to be in the world, the more we forget ourselves the greater our chance at actualization. The more we are outer directed in terms of what we may give to others, the greater the chance for actualization.

Frankl's theory of logotherapy is future oriented in that he speaks of the necessity of looking at a purpose to be fulfilled in the future. According to Frankl, "A man who becomes conscious of the responsibility he bears toward a human being who affectionately waits for him, or to an unfinished work, will never throw away his life. He knows the "why" for his existence, and will be able to bear almost any "how"."[8]

Lastly, Frankl brings in the past into focus because he also speaks in such a way that honors the past:

> What you have experienced, no power on earth can take from you. Not only your experiences, but all we have done, whatever great thoughts we may have had, and all we have suffered, all this is not lost, though it is past; we

6 Frankl, 111–112.
7 Frankl, 111.
8 Frankl, 80.

have brought it into being. Having been is also a kind of being, and perhaps the surest kind.[9]

Therefore, I think Frankl is saying that we need to establish a balance within our own minds regarding the past, the present, and the future. We need to pay attention to all three and not focus our attention exclusively on one. I think that the trick to master is to live in all three tenses simultaneously.

Frankl speaks about how the loss of hope is the precursor of death. He talks about not only the psychological effects of a loss of hope can have but of the physiological effects the loss of hope can have as well. He writes about a friend of his within the camps who had a dream that liberation would come by a certain day (March 13th) and when liberation did not come on that day, his health took a turn for the worse. He was dead by March 31st. Frankl writes:

> Those who know how close the connection is between the state of mind of a man—his courage and hope, or lack of them—and the state of immunity of his body will understand that the sudden loss of hope and courage can have a deadly effect. The ultimate loss of hope and courage was that the expected liberation did not come and he was severely disappointed. This suddenly lowered his body's resistance against the latest typhus infection. His faith in the future and his will to live had become paralyzed and his body fell victim to illness—and thus the voice of his dream was right after all.[10]

Frankl writes about how his desire to once again see his wife and his desire to write his book are what led to his survival. His future book saved his life in more than one way. He came into the camp with his manuscript sown into the lining of his coat, but his coat was taken from him upon entry. He writes about the despondency he felt upon losing the manuscript, but he decided that he would live his thoughts in the present instead of writing them. He writes of the experience like this:

> Instead of the many pages of my manuscript, I found in a pocket of the newly acquired coat one single page torn out a Hebrew prayer book, containing the

9 Frankl, 82.
10 Frankl, 75.

> most important Jewish prayer, Shema Yisrael. How should I have interpreted such a "coincidence" other than as a challenge to live my thoughts instead of merely putting them on paper?[11]

He also writes about reconstructing the book within his mind, by looking back and remembering is what saved his life as well. When he was ill with typhus fever, he jotted down notes that he could remember from his old manuscript, and he states that he was convinced that reconstruction was what helped him to overcome the danger of cardiovascular collapse.[12]

He writes about imagining himself as a person with a future was another strategy used to preserve his life:

> I forced my thoughts to turn to another subject. Suddenly I saw myself standing on the platform of a well-lit, warm and pleasant lecture room. In front of me sat an attentive audience on comfortable upholstered seats. I was giving a lecture on the psychology of the concentration camp! All that oppressed me at that moment became objective, seen and described from the remote viewpoint of science. By this method I succeeded somehow in rising above the situation, above the sufferings of the moment, and I observed them as if they were already in the past.[13]

This passage is so interesting for several reasons. One, he is using his imagination to see what direction his work may take him in the future. Two, he is developing a purely objective stance toward his current situation and envisioning how it may become useful in the future. Three, he uses the objective stance to allow him to rise about his current condition. Developing objectivity is one strategy that Frankl uses to help him survive. The other strategy Frankl tells us is essential is developing a sense of humor.[14] Humor, when seen within this context, may be seen as its own form of objectivity. In order to see humor within our situations, it requires that we detach a bit and to not take everything so personally.

11 Frankl, 115.
12 Frankl, 104.
13 Frankl, 73.
14 Frankl, 43 & 44.

Of humor, Frankl writes: "Humor was another of the soul's weapons in the fight for self-preservation."[15]

Frankl both embodies and writes about the concept of self-actualization or the moving forward in life toward what one should become. In using the language of actualization, Frankl is, once again, evoking the work of Abraham Masow. Frankl makes clear that actualization is an ongoing process and therefore it has no end point. According to Frankl:

> I never tire of saying that the only really transitory aspects of life are the potentialities; but as soon as they are actualized, they are rendered realities at that very moment; they are saved and delivered into the past, wherein they are rescued and preserved from transitoriness. For, in the past, nothing is irretrievably lost but everything irrevocably stored.[16]

Here, Frankl lays out for us how the three tenses inform one another. Even though the theory of logotherapy places an emphasis on the future, it never does so at the expense of the present and past. Frankl's entire book is about what potential the present provides us.

It is all about how we choose to respond to the present moment but that responsibility entails remembering the past and planning for the future as well. In the next chapter, I will address the capacity to rise above life's circumstances as well as the philosopher who was the inspiration for Frankl's ideal.

References

Frankl, Viktor E. *Man's Search for Meaning.* Boston: Beacon Press, 2006.

Goethe, Johann Wolfgang von. *Wilhelm Meister's Apprentice.* Kalamazoo, MI: River Run Press, 1982. Book 8.

15 Frankl, 43.

16 Frankl, 120.

Chapter Six

The Uberman

The philosopher Friederich Nietzsche played a major role within Frankl's book. I would even go so far to say that Frankl could not have written the book without knowing of the work of Nietzsche. In fact, one of the famous quotes attributed to Frankl is not Frankl but Nietzsche: "He who has a *why* to live for can bear with almost any *how*."[1] Frankl built his entire theory of logotherapy around this Nietzschean idea of purpose.

Frankl says that the above quote originates with Nietzsche while other times, he is writing about a Nietzschean concept without using Nietzsche's words. Nietzsche wrote about the uberman or the man who rises above. Frankl writes about those who are capable of rising above. If we look at Frankl's words, he tells us: "Yet one of the main features of human existence is the capacity to rise above such conditions, to grow beyond them."[2] And sometimes he speaks of rising above using more Nietzschean language: "For what matters is to bear witness to the

1 Frankl, 76.
2 Frankl, 131.

uniquely human potential at its best, which is to transform a personal tragedy into a human achievement."[3]

This last statement conveys the Nietzschean ideal, and it fits in with Frankl's Stoic understanding of transforming suffering into a gift. When I talk to students about Frankl's concept of rising above, we can most definitely use Frankl's life as an example. Frankl was the uberman within his own life but there are others as well. I teach my students about the concentration camp survivor, Eva Moses Kor. Moses Kor was captured, as a child, by the Nazis and suffered extreme torture at the hands of the Nazis because she and her sister were twins. The Nazis had a morbid fascination with twins and conducted horrific experimentations on them. Moses Kor and her sister were no different. Both managed to survive and when Moses Kor's sister died as an adult, many years later, it was discovered that her internal organs never matured as she grew because of the experimentation she was subjected to within the camps. Moses Kor decided to write a letter of forgiveness to a former Nazi SS member. She then decided to deliver that letter. She talks about how she thought that act of forgiveness was for him, but the act of forgiveness ended up being for herself.

What Moses Kor discovers through her own experience is the embodiment of how Frankl speaks of actualizing one's own potential. In Frankl's words:

> By declaring that man is responsible and must actualize the potential meaning of his life, I wish to stress that the true meaning of life is to be discovered in the world rather than within man or his own psyche, as though it were a closed system. I have termed this constitutive characteristic "the self-transcendence of human existence." It denotes the fact that being human always points, and is directed, to something, or someone, other than oneself—be it a meaning to fulfill or another human being to encounter. The more one forgets himself—by giving himself to a cause to serve or another person to love—the more human he is and the more he actualizes himself.[4]

Frankl is consistently telling us that we reach our potential by reaching out. We do not reach our potential without giving to another. The

3 Frankl, 112.
4 Frankl, 110–111.

giving must be done freely, expecting nothing in return. This part of the book connects us to Frankl's claim that our highest purpose is love or agape. The more we choose to live in love and through love, the more human we become and the greatest opportunity we have of living up to our potential.

The next part of this argument, Frankl makes clear that self-transcendence is not a reachable goal because like success, the more we make it a product, the more we miss it. In other words, we move toward self-actualization by forgetting about ourselves and giving to others because we can. Let's read Frankl's words:

> What is called self-actualization is not an attainable aim at all, for the simple reason that the more one would strive for it, the more he would miss it. In other words, self-actualization is possible only as a side-effect of self-transcendence.[5]

The focus of this book is how we can create a life that is meaningful. We have been examining how we can decide to create a life worth living. Frankl is telling us that we cannot create this life sitting in a room alone. It requires that we move out into the world to understand what we have to offer. It may sound hackneyed, but this gives meaning to the expression that if you can, no matter how seemingly small, try to give to others. I realize that if you are depressed, the idea of giving to others may sound insurmountable but it does not need to be a grand gesture. We may find that reaching out to another and making connections to lift someone's spirits unintentionally ends up lifting our own spirits.

Frankl states that self-actualization is a never attainable goal because it is a process. Once something has been achieved, we need to move forward. We are never done but instead an ongoing work-in-progress. According to Frankl:

> I never tire of saying that the only really transitory aspects of life are the potentialities; but as soon as they are actualized they are rendered realities at that very moment; they are saved and delivered into the past, wherein they

5 Frankl, 111.

> are rescued and preserved from transitoriness. For, in the past, nothing is irretrievably lost but everything irrevocably stored.[6]

Frankl is working with the Nietzschean ideal of the uberman (although he never uses that word) to address how we decide to interact with the circumstances we find ourselves. The Nietzschean ideal of the uberman is connected to Frankl's critique of pan-determinism:

> By that I mean the view of man which disregards his capacity to take a stand toward any conditions whatsoever. Man is not fully conditioned and determined but rather determines himself whether he gives in to conditions or stands up to them. In other words, man is ultimately self-determining. Man does not simply exist but always decides what his existence will be, what he will become in the next moment.[7]

This description of self-determination will sound consistent with a Stoic/existential view of man. Given that man is radically free, he is then free to make whatever he chooses from his life circumstances. According to this philosophy, we cannot change the circumstances of our lives, but we are free as to how to see the circumstances. Within this context, I would like to return once again to the story of Eva Moses Kor, who through the eyes of some was "scathingly condemned as a scandalous traitor to her people."[8] In calling her a traitor, her freedom is being taken from her yet again. The philosophical tradition that Frankl uses within his book places Moses Kor's decision within the realm of her own life. She does not need to be who her community expects her to be. I have seen this happen in other contexts as well. Sometimes groups are perceived as monoliths and any action or word spoken that is not in accordance with the group is perceived as going against the group. There have been other public stories that also had to do with forgiveness where the individual was seen as a traitor to his/her community by choosing to forgive.[9] According to the perspective offered here, we

6 Frankl, 120.
7 Frankl, 131.
8 https://plus61j.net.au/editors-picks/holocaust-survivor-forgiveness-ultimate-revenge/
9 Brandt Jean, (in 2019) brother of Botham Jean, forgave the police officer who shot and killed his brother. Also, Kathrine Switzer (in 1967) became friends with the

are accountable to ourselves for our choices because we are free, and we alone are responsible for our choices.

These ubermen are well-known within the public domain but I have had ubermen and women within my classes. One student, Shylove, had a job within an assisted living facility. She arrived one morning to take care of an elderly bed-ridden woman. The older woman said to my student: "I do not want any N-word taking care of me." My student responded: "I am happy to be an N-word and I am happy to take care of you." Shylove, in my opinion, is the epitome of the uberman. She rose above her circumstance. She did not react to the woman but instead stayed true to herself. As these things frequently develop, after the older woman saw that Shylove was not going anywhere and took very good care of the woman, the woman only wanted to be cared for by Shylove. We can see examples of the uberman within our everyday life and I frequently see these qualities within my students.

One final point about the Nietzschean concept of the uberman is that Hitler appropriated the concept and transformed the idea into the Aryan ideal. This was not Nietzsche's intention. The uberman was the result of an internal struggle and the individual's discipline to overcome. It was not a birthright of a superior nationality. In the hands of Hitler, the Nietzschean ideal was transformed into a racist agenda. This could be one of the reasons why Frankl does not use the term within his book. The term itself is controversial because of what it became. A similar fate surrounded what we now call the Nazi swastika. The symbol was present in many different cultures as the symbol of well-being. Some theories postulate that nineteenth century German scholars who translated old Indian texts noticed similarities between their own language and Sanskrit. This was the beginning of the appropriation of the symbol to signify a race of white god-like people called Aryans.

On a trip to the island of Cyprus, I remember seeing the symbol on one floor mosaic of an ancient Cypriot home. The meaning, within that context, was one of well-being or good fortune. The symbol can never

Boston Marathon director, John Duncan "Jock" Semple, who attacked her during the race because he did not know that a female had registered to run the race. She had registered using only her initials and up until then, only one other woman (Bobbi Gibb in 1966) had competed.

return to that pre-Nazi meaning. It is a crime to display a swastika in Germany and I remember reading a story about a German woman who baked a swastika into a cake and was arrested when she posted the picture on social media. In the US, display of the Nazi swastika is protected as free speech but as the case of Germany shows us, a different history gives rise to different laws.

So much of how we choose to behave comes down to how we choose to see the other. The Nazi saw himself as superior to the Jew. The older woman saw my student as less than because of skin color. My student, however, did not return hate with hate but instead returned hate with love. That is why I write about her as the uberman. In the next chapter, I will explore some of the nuances of how we see the other and how this topic is presented within Frankl's work.

References

Borschel-Dan, Amada. "Holocaust Survivor Preaches Forgiveness of Nazis as Ultimate Revenge," *The Times of Israel.* 8 December 2016. https://plus61j.net.au/editors-picks/holocaust-survivor-forgiveness-ultimate-revenge/

Frankl, Viktor E. *Man's Search for Meaning.* Boston: Beacon Press, 2006.

Chapter Seven

The Other

Frankl is telling us that our highest purpose in life is to give to others. The question then becomes: how is it that we choose to see the other? We can see the other through the eyes of love or through a darker lens that manifests in feelings such as hatred, revenge, or blame. The word we can begin with to understand our relationship with others is the word host. We serve as hosts to each other. The word host is ambiguous, and that ambiguity is important because it tells us that how we see the other is our choice. Host can mean someone who receives guests, and this meaning is conveyed in the words hospitality, hospital, and hostel. The word can also mean enemy as conveyed in the words hostage and hostility. The word host could also refer to the eucharist and signify the body and blood of Jesus Christ. Host may refer to someone officiating a gathering, harboring the enemy, or receiving communion. The ambiguity tells us that it is our choice whether we see the other as friend, enemy, or godly and the choice has to do with how we see ourselves. We typically project onto others what belongs to ourselves.

I have earlier quoted from a beautiful essay on the power of the spoken word by Diane Glancy who tells us: "You kept in mind that what the speaker says affects the speaker as much as the spoken to."[1] One is free to create misery for others but in doing so, one is creating misery for oneself. Passing on one's abuse that one has been subjected to is to recreate the abuse for oneself. It doesn't much matter that you are now the abuser instead of the abused. Frankl addresses the complexity of the cyclical nature of abuse when he speaks about how some prisoners, upon release, recreated the abuse that they once were subjected to. He calls this type of person "primitive" and identifies that they lacked the discipline of mind to let go of the brutality which had surrounded them in camp life. Frankl tells us that the only difference was they were now the oppressors instead of the oppressed. "They became instigators, not objects, of willful force and injustice. They justified their behavior by their own terrible experience."[2]

To once again return to the philosophical foundations of the book is to return to the notion that we are all free to make our own choices. We can, of course, be free to reinforce the status quo and do unto others the same bad things that have been done unto us. This, though, is to participate in the recreation of our own hell. Frankl is correct in calling this a primitive reaction and we need to ask ourselves to have the presence of mind to create something that better serves everyone's best interest. Frankl cautions about the bitterness that could eat away at some of the former prisoners upon release:

> A friend was walking across a field with me toward a camp when suddenly we came to a field of green crops. Automatically, I avoided it, but he drew his arm through mine and dragged me through it. I stammered something about not treading on the young crops. He became annoyed, gave me an angry look and shouted, "You don't say! And hasn't enough been taken from us? My wife and child have been gassed—not to mention everything else—and you would forbid me to tread on a few stalks of oats!"[3]

Of course, the backdrop of Frankl's book is that an entire community of people agreed to scapegoat the Jews. The term scapegoat is

1 Diane Glancy, "Speaking the Corn into Being," in *The West Pole* (Minneapolis: University of Minnesota Press, 1997).
2 Frankl, 90.
3 Frankl, 90.

Biblical, and it referred to an actual goat. The high priest would hold up a goat and ask the people to transfer their sins to the animal and then the animal would be slaughtered thereby absolving the people of their sins. Two characteristics are most certainly always true of scapegoats—they are usually a powerless, disenfranchised group and the search for the scapegoat is usually when events have taken a steep decline downward. I have taught Frankl's book for a very long time, and I have seen different groups move into the position of scapegoat. Moving different groups of people into the lower rung of the social hierarchy is no change. Dismantling the need for the creation of the scapegoat would be a change and taking responsibility for conditions would also be a desirable change.

The scapegoat, used within interpersonal and political contexts, serves to avoid the kind of introspection and responsibility that leads to self-empowerment. The creation of scapegoats serves to maintain the status quo within the culture. Nothing fundamentally changes because all that we do not wish to see within ourselves is projected onto the scapegoat. Their symbolic or actual death is the purification of the sins we do not wish to acknowledge within ourselves.

Hitler gained political traction by the creation of the Jew as scapegoat. Unfortunately, we seemingly have learned little from history because the creation of the scapegoat is very much alive within America. Just as the bully, within the interpersonal context, is unwell so it also true within a national context. The person or the country seeking a scapegoat as the receptacle for all that they wish to discard is a red flag for a lack of self-worth. Bullies behave the way that they do because they are broken and rather than acknowledging their brokenness, they attempt to project their brokenness onto others. I invite my students to read an article called "Sing Your Song" that speaks about African tribal wisdom: "The tribe understood that the correction for antisocial behavior is love and the remembrance of identity."[4] In response to wrong-doing, the child was encircled by the elders as they reminded him of their love and held out the option for the child to do better. This tribal wisdom seemed to be the foundational thinking for the movement of restorative justice. This

4 Alan Cohen, "Sing Your Song," *Wisdom of the Heart* (New York: Hay House, 2002), 4–5.

article offers the message that expelling the bully from the community may be the opposite of what is needed. By pushing away the bully, we may be strengthening the bullying. We need to embrace the bully, as difficult as that may be, and attempt to bring him back into the community. This is especially true when the bully is a child.

The larger point that Frankl is making here is that we as a species need to get off this hamster wheel that we have constructed with the creation of the scapegoat and the search for revenge by those who have been scapegoated. The creation of the scapegoat never absolves the creator of responsibility and the desire for destruction and revenge never makes the person harmed feel better. When looked at within this frame, the lust for revenge is to lose oneself in the world the enemy has created. Frankl never speaks of seeking revenge upon the Nazis because then the Nazis would have won. Nelson Mandela provided us with the same lesson that Frankl is offering. Once released from prison and elected as President of South African, Mandela was said to be having lunch with his security guards at a restaurant where he spotted one of his former jailors also eating lunch. He invited the man to join them for lunch. The man was visibly shaken because the jailor had subjected Mandela to torture while under his guard.[5] Mandela, like Frankl, advocated that compassion and love are qualities that compose human nature and humanity would be able to advance in this way if people were not taught hate and fear. It sounds like a cliche to say these statements but not when backed up with the life experiences of people like Frankl and Mandela who had every reason to seek revenge and instead chose not to hate.

The desire for revenge always points to something missing within ourselves and the search for revenge is futile. The writer George Orwell writes about his witnessing an encounter between a former S.S. officer and a Jew. Here is what this encounter sounds like in the hands of Orwell:

5 Stephanie Nolen, "Mandela's Miraculous Capacity for Forgiveness: A Carefully Calibrated Strategy," *The Globe and Mail*, 5 December 2013. https://www.theglobeandmail.com/news/world/nelson-mandela-miraculous-capacity-for-forgiveness-a-carefully-calibrated-strategy/article548192.

> It is absurd to blame any German or Austrian Jew for getting his own back on the Nazi. Heaven knows what scores this particular man may have had to wipe out: very likely his whole family had been murdered; and, after all, a wanton kick to a prisoner is a very tiny thing compared with the outrages committed by the Hitler regime. But what this scene, and much else that I saw in Germany, brought home to me was that the whole idea of revenge and punishment is a childish day-dream. Properly speaking there is no such thing as revenge. Revenge is an act which you want to commit when you are powerless and because you are powerless: as soon as the sense of impotence is removed, the desire evaporates also.[6]

Frankl and Mandela both embody the insight that Orwell offers. These were men who had no use for revenge because they both had power. The kind of power they had was true power that comes in the form of personal power within one's life. Their power was not the imitation of power that looms over others that is often mistaken for power but instead both these men made up their minds that, in spite of the brutality directed toward them, they would choose another path. Both men left us with evidence that it can be done and, in their writings, left us a blueprint on how to do it.

Within the next chapter, I will further explore Frankl's choice not to grow bitter because he suffered greatly during his imprisonment.

References

Cohen, Alan. "Sing Your Song," in *Wisdom of the Heart*. New York: Hay House, 2002.

Glancy, Diane. "Speaking the Corn into Being," in *The West Pole*. Minneapolis, MN: 1999. Also, *Utne Reader*, 1 September 1997. https://utne.com/mind-and-body/speaking-the-corn-into-being-cherokee-oral-tradition

Nolan, Stephanie. "Mandela's Miraculous Capacity for Forgiveness: A Carefully Calibrated Strategy," *The Globe and Mail*, 5 December 2013. https://www.theglobeandmail.com/news/world/nelson-mandela-miraculous-capacity-for-forgiveness-a-carefully-calibrated-strategy/article548192

Orwell, George. "Revenge is Sour," in *Facing Unpleasant Facts*. Boston: Mariner Books, 2008, 184–188.

6 George Orwell, "Revenge is Sour," in *Facing Unpleasant Facts: Narrative Essays* (Boston: Mariner Books, 2008), 186.

Chapter Eight

Tragic Optimism

Toward the end of the book, Frankl writes about what he calls "a case for tragic optimism."[1] I would like to focus on these words to make several points about what Frankl is telling us. The first observation, of course, is that the phrase is an oxymoron. Life is clearly tragic in that bad things happen and all life entails death. As I get older, the reality that we do not get to live forever gets to become so much more of a reality. This is especially true when one is a parent and even more so when is a parent of a child with special needs. The thought of leaving this world and leaving behind my son is sometimes more than I can bear. The existential reality is, of course, tragic but the choice to remain optimistic is also infinitely practical. When Frankl talks about life being tragic and the choice to remain optimistic despite it all is wise and it is the wisdom he inherited from the Stoics. Sure, we can choose a more pessimistic way of going through life but that would only create bad outcomes for both ourselves and those around us. A choice to be

1 Frankl, 137.

optimistic, on the other hand, is life-affirming and reinforces the choice to move forward.

Frankl writes of the importance of letting go of the bad things that have happened to us because if we do not, we remain stuck in the past and forever identified with the previous harm. In the previous chapter, I wrote about a woman who chose to forgive the Nazis for the crimes they committed. She was under the impression that the act of forgiveness was for the Nazi but she discovered that in the end, it was for her. The act of forgiveness released her from what was done in the past. A similar notion applies to the self in that if we do not forgive ourselves for what we did in the past, we are forever connected and tied back to one act. The philosopher Hannah Arendt,as usual, got it right:

> Without being forgiven, released from the consequences of what we have done, our capacity to act would, as it were, be confined to one single deed from which we would never recover; we would remain the victims of its consequences forever, not unlike the sorcerer's apprentice who lacked the formula to break the spell.[2]

I have shared this quote with many students over the years because I think Arendt captures the capacity to become stuck and how a lack of forgiveness inhibits our capacity to act in the world.

In the previous chapter, I discussed the scene in the book where the former prisoner unconsciously destroys crops under his feet because he feels entitled to now become destructive based on what he has had to endure in the past. I think that this mentality is very common, and it is what prevents people from moving forward and creating a better life. In addition to the Stoic roots present within Frankl's concept of tragic optimism, I think it also connects with another ancient concept that I learned while I was an undergraduate.

Epideictic rhetoric was defined by Aristotle as speech of praise or blame.[3]

2 Hannah Arendt, *The Human Condition* (Chicago: The University of Chicago Press, 1958), 237.

3 For a discussion of how I came to think about epideictic see Janet Farrell Leontiou, *Food for Thought: The Rhetoric of Babette's Feast.* Unpublished dissertation, Penn State University 1994.

Epideictic, though, was more than a type of speech but it was, instead, a way of being. According to my teacher, Lawrence W. Rosenfield:

> I contend, in brief, that we misconstrue epideictic when we hold it fundamental tactics to praise and blame. What is involved instead may be more accurately thought of as "acknowledgment" and "disparagement," the recognition of what is (goodness, grace, intrinsic excellence) or the refusal to so recognize in a moment of inspiration. In either case the experience afforded the participants is the opportunity of beholding reality impartially as a witness of Being.[4]

When I read this statement, I see so much common ground between epideictic, stoicism, and logotherapy. In each context, there is the wisdom of saying "yes" to life. Bitterness and complaint is really antithetical to life because it says that how things are is not good enough. I learned as an undergraduate in communication classes that appreciation is a choice and the more I start to see what is right in front of me, the more I can respond with appreciation. Like everything else when I change how I look, I change what I see. This is especially true when we come to speak about what we find to be beautiful. I love what the Irish writer, John O'Donohue, states about beauty:

> We have often heard that beauty is in the eye of the beholder. This is usually taken to mean that the sense of beauty is utterly subjective; there is no accounting for taste because each person's taste is different. The statement has another, more subtle meaning: if our style of looking becomes beautiful, then beauty will become visible and shine forth for us. We will be surprised to discover beauty in unexpected places where the ungraceful eye would never linger. The graced eye can glimpse beauty anywhere, for beauty does not reserve itself for special elite moments or instances; it does not wait for perfection but is present already secretly in everything. When we beautify our gaze, the grace of hidden beauty becomes our joy and sanctuary.[5]

4 Lawrence W. Rosenfield, "The Practical Celebration of Epideictic," in *Rhetoric in Transition: Studies in the Nature and Uses of Rhetoric* ed. Eugene E. White (University Park: The Pennsylvania State University Press, 1980), 133.

5 John O'Donohue, *Beauty: The Invisible Embrace* (New York: Harper Perennial, 2005), 19.

I remember learning from reading the philosophy of Gadamer that objectivity is attaining the truth regarding the object, and I think that O'Donohue is expressing a similar point of view. Objectivity is being able to see what is or as Rosenfield would say the ability "of beholding reality impartially."

Part of the development of my theory of logostherapy is to learn to attend to words objectively. When I attend to the etymology of a word objectively, I learn the truth of the word.

When I attend to the words of others, I try to understand the truth of what they are saying and the same goes for attending to my own words. I try to develop the objectivity to understand if my words are offered out of habit or, instead, from genuine intention. I can also listen to the presence of words of complaint, gossip, and put downs versus the words of acceptance, friendship and celebration. To be sure, there is lots of normalized negativity present expressed through language within our culture and we need to start to understand that these words will never lift us up but instead always bring us down. I think that many within the culture suffer from a depletion of energy but may not be aware that this is the result of feeding on a steady diet of negativity both in the words listened to and produced.

Frankl identifies developing objectivity as one way to master the art of living. The other essential quality to possess, according to Frankl, is having a sense of humor. We can immediately see that both objectivity and humor are closely related. Humor is the ability to detach a bit and not take everything that happens to us so personally. According to Frankl:

> Humor was another of the soul's weapons in the fight for self-preservation. It is well known that humor, more than anything else in the human make-up, can afford an aloofness and an ability to rise above any situation, even if only for a few seconds.[6]

In this passage, Frankl is telling us how essential it is to have a sense of humor and how a sense of humor may play a role in becoming an uberman within our own lives. The physical quality of the uberman is

6 Frankl, 43.

a twinkle in their eye. Frankl, as seen on YouTube archive video, had it. Moses Kor had it. Both had so much taken from them by the Nazis, but they did not allow the Nazis to rob them of their spirits.

The important point that Frankl reminds us to carry with us is not to give in to despair.

The ancient mentality also understood the importance of celebrating all that has been given. They understood that it is precisely that which makes life most challenging and difficult is that which causes us to grow in ways we could not imagine without the suffering serving as the catalyst. Frankl talks about those people who suffer from "give-up-itis"[7] as suffering from a forgetfulness: "Such people forget that often it is such an exceptionally difficult external situation which gives man the opportunity to grow spiritually beyond himself."[8] He is telling us to be patient and allow the meaning of the experience to be revealed to us. We only construct meaning by looking back. We often do not know the significance of something while we are having the experience. Meaning is constructed by holding the experience within our memory and engaging in retrospect. He provides us with the hopeful perspective, based upon his clinical work, that people who had attempted suicide and failed were later relieved of the failed attempt. According to Frankl:

> I explain to such a person that patients have repeatedly told me how happy they were that the suicide attempt had not been successful; weeks, months, years later, they told me, it turned out that there *was* a solution to their problem, an answer to their question, a meaning to their life.[9]

In order to get to this place of gratitude, however, one must hold on in order that she or he live to see it. I know that the reason that someone chooses to take his or her life is that the pain has become too great to bear. However, the choice to end one's pain is always simultaneously the choice to prolong someone else's pain. Those who are left behind will never experience an end to the pain of having lost their beloved.

7 Frankl, 139.
8 Frankl, 72.
9 Frankl, 142.

That was why I was taken by my student's comment that the thought of my student's mother is what saved her life. I do not think that my student understood the profound connection she had at that moment. Becoming outwardly directed saved her life.

Life is tragic, as Frankl tells us, but we need to develop an optimistic state of mind.

At the end of the book, Frankl offers a story of a man who, through an accident, became a quadriplegic. Frankl offers us the man's words: "I view my life as being abundant with meaning and purpose. The attitude that I adopted on that fateful day has become my personal credo for life: I broke my neck, it didn't break me."[10] I love this quote because I think that Jerry Long embodies the habit of mind Frankl is speaking about. The word *optimism* comes from Ops, who in Roman mythology, was the deity of abundance. Long makes clear that this is not something that happens automatically but is instead the result of the choice to see one's life as abundantly meaningful.

References

Arendt, Hannah. *The Human Condition.* Chicago: The University of Chicago Press, 1958.

Farrell Leontiou, Janet. "Food for Thought: The Rhetoric of Babette's Feast." Unpublished Ph.D. dissertation. Penn State University, 1994.

Frankl, Viktor E. *Man's Search for Meaning.* Boston: Beacon Press, 2006.

O'Donohue, John. *Beauty: The Invisible Embrace.* New York: Harper Perennial, 2005.

Rosenfield, L.W. "The Practical Celebration of Epideictic," in *Rhetoric in Translation: Studies in The Nature and Uses of Rhetoric.* Eugene E. White (ed.). University Park: Penn State University Press, 1980, 131–155.

10 Frankl, 147.

Conclusion

In this book, I hope that I have added some value to Frankl's theory of logotherapy. I have tried to make the argument that all words have roots or ancestry as well as wings or legacy. The roots that I have stressed throughout are the connections of logotherapy to Stoicism. I do not think that these roots are particularly stressed within Frankl's book and the connections are only present within one preface of one edition of the book.[1] I think that by understanding logotherapy's roots in Stoicism, makes it a richer theory. By stressing the interrelatedness of the Stoic ideas of acceptance, responsibility, freedom, and of course the power of the logos has us see that Frankl's theory of logotherapy is both a moving forward and a returning back.

The legacy of logotherapy is what has allowed me to formulate a theory of logostherapy. This theory allows us, I hope, to go deeper into the three ways in which we create meaning in our lives. Understanding the etymology of love, work, and suffering allows us to more fully

1 Preface written by Gordon W. Allport in Viktor E. Frankl, *Man's Search for Meaning* (New York: Simon & Schuster, Inc., 1959), 9–13.

understand how Frankl wished for us to conceive of these aspects of our lives. A focus on words also allows us to more fully grasp Frankl's meaning throughout the book. I have also attempted to offer examples throughout for us to think about what our own words are doing.

Frankl is writing within the field of psychology that is strongly influenced by philosophy. I am, instead, writing within the field of communication. Frankl states that one of the reasons for the book's success is because we are in desperate need of its message.[2] I also think that one of the main reasons why we experience the state of meaninglessness that we do is because we have lost the understanding of the power of the word. I would go so far to say that we cannot have a meaningful life if we look upon words as meaningless. My work over the last twenty-seven years has been to uncover this awareness of the power of the word.

The word philosophy is Greek, and it means the lover or friend of wisdom. One of the reasons why Frankl was able to survive the camps was because he carried the ancient Stoic wisdom with him. I worry for my students because more and more, we live within a world that values that which is current above all else and that sometimes results in a lack of appreciation for ancient wisdom. In teaching my students about the Stoics, it is my wish that their ideas are also able to save my students' lives as well. Although there is no comparison between what Frankl experienced and the lives of my students, I do worry about the existential abyss impacting so many of them.

At times, it was difficult to write the individual chapters of this book because the topics are all interrelated and feed into one another. Frankl's *Man's Search for Meaning* ends with "A Case for Tragic Optimism." As I noted earlier, I read this part of the book as a nod to what the ancients would have called epideictic rhetoric. An epideictic framework, consistent with Stoicism, emphasizes celebration, thoughtfulness, memory, choice, and gratitude. Gratitude not just for some aspects of life but for all of it. And as I learned from my teacher, Larry Rosenfield, gratitude is not a response to a deed already done but instead a state of readiness and a way of being in the world. I think that this is the reason why I was immediately drawn to Frankl's work. Frankl, like Rosenfield, worked

2 Frankl, xiii.

on carrying the message to us to engage in a metanoia (a complete change of mind) recognized by the ancients as the superior way to live.

My work in writing this book was not to survey the academic landscape to see what scholars have said about Frankl's work. Instead, I attempted to write about how I have worked with these ideas over the last twenty-seven years because I have seen that the way I have attempted to breathe new life into Frankl's ideas has been effective in reaching an audience of students. I wrote the book with the hope of expanding that immediate audience.

At the end of the book, Frankl recounts his words to First World Congress of Logotherapy in 1980: "I argued not only for the rehumanization of psychology but also for what I called 'the Degurufication of logotherapy.' My interest does not lie in raising parrots that just rehash 'their Master's voice,' but rather in passing the torch to 'independent and inventive, innovative and creative spirits.'"[3] I sincerely wish that Frankl would think that I have made a contribution to his work, and I hope that he would have been pleased to know that I have devoted my professional career to bringing his work to community college students. Many students over the years have used what they have learned to launch their lives in new directions. I have written about how one group of community college students, as inspired by reading Frankl and learning about the Stoics, created their own theory—a theory on listening. Sitting in that classroom listening to my students present their theory to the class is a day I will never forget. I have now written this book with the same intention extended to my readers. I hope that as you have read this book, you have been inspired to breathe new life into these very old ideas and you then carry these ideas to a world that very much needs them. I end with Frankl's poignant words: "For the world is in a bad state, but everything will become still worse unless each of us does his best."[4] To do one's best is to choose to live up to one's potential and to live up to one's potential always entails reaching outward.

3 Frankl, 153.
4 Frankl, 154.

Health Communication

Gary L. Kreps, Series Editor

This series examines the powerful influences of human and mediated communication in delivering care and promoting health.

Books analyze the ways that strategic communication humanizes and increases access to quality care as well as examining the use of communication to encourage pro-active health promotion. The books describe strategies for addressing major health issues, such as reducing health disparities, minimizing health risks, responding to health crises, encouraging early detection and care, facilitating informed health decisionmaking, promoting coordination within and across health teams, overcoming health literacy challenges, designing responsive health information technologies, and delivering sensitive end-of-life care.

All books in the series are grounded in broad evidence-based scholarship and are vivid, compelling, and accessible to broad audiences of scholars, students, professionals, and laypersons.

For additional information about this series or for the submission of manuscripts, please contact:

Gary L. Kreps
University Distinguished Professor and Chair, Department of Communication
Director, Center for Health and Risk Communication
George Mason University Science & Technology 2, Suite 230, MS 3D6
Fairfax, VA 22030-4444
gkreps@gmu.edu

To order other books in this series, please contact our Customer Service Department:

peterlang@presswarehouse.com (within the U.S.)
orders@peterlang.com (outside the U.S.)

Or browse online by series:
www.peterlang.com

www.ingramcontent.com/pod-product-compliance
Ingram Content Group UK Ltd.
Pitfield, Milton Keynes, MK11 3LW, UK
UKHW021010120926
8556IPUK00029B/444